NUTRITION AND ATHLETIC PERFORMANCE

Edited by
WILLIAM HASKELL, Ph.D.
JAMES SCALA, P
JAMES WHITTAM, P

Proceedings of the
Conference on Nutritional Determinants
in Athletic Performance
San Francisco, California
September 24-25, 1981

Designer: Lois Stanfield

Copyright 1982 by Bull Publishing Company,
P.O. Box 208 Palo Alto, California 94302.

ISBN 0-915950-56-1

Table of Contents

Introduction

This Symposium, Nutritional Determinants in Athletic Performance, was organized for the exchange of scientific information on how to improve the performance and health of participants in vigorous, competitive exercise. The program was specifically designed to provide a "state of the science" review for coaches, trainers, dietitians, teachers and physicians responsible for the training and care of athletes.

A secondary, but no less important, objective was to provide an opportunity for scientists in medicine, nutrition, biochemistry and physiology to exchange information on new study results and methods— to question old and newly accepted nutrition and performance-related practices; and to propose priorities for future research. It also provided an opportunity for an enthusiastic and informative exchange of ideas concerning the roles of nutrition, fluid intake, and body composition on athletic performance, and of some of the special nutritional considerations for the younger, older, diabetic and female athlete.

The issues addressed in this Symposium relate to the fundamental principles of nutrition and athletic performance, as they are currently understood. While much new information has been developed during the past decade, due to intensive research and new improved means of measurement, the data demonstrate the old scientific adage, "the more you learn, the more you need to know." This Symposium raised as many questions as it answered—which potentially is productive, if it leads to the development, dissemination and use of new information. From our perspective, this is a positive approach, as it does much to focus on key issues which need further scientific consideration.

Finally, we feel the interaction that occurs, when members from various disciplines in the scientific community get together to share their own unique knowledge and experiences, is essential for solving the issues in sports medicine. The athlete, coach, trainer and sports physician provide the real-life practical problems and case studies; the physiologist, biochemist and other scientists measure the effects, and propose solutions, and the nutritionist or dietitian provide the mechanism for implementing the solutions. All are essential for a satisfactory response to the challenge of developing nutritional guidelines for optimizing health and performance. This Symposium was an important step in that direction.

The Proceedings have been organized in a very straightforward format. The manuscripts presented at each session were reviewed, edited, and in some cases updated and published here as the foundation for each topic discussed at the Symposium. At the end of each section we have presented a summary of the major issues addressed during the discussion sessions. Our goal was simply to identify relevant issues, not to draw conclusions.

William L. Haskell, Ph.D.
Stanford University

James H. Whittam, Ph.D.
Shaklee Corporation

James Scala, Ph.D.
Shaklee Corporation

SUBSTRATE UTILIZATION AND ATHLETIC PERFORMANCE

Fats, Carbohydrates, and Protein: Why We Need Them, And How They Are Obtained

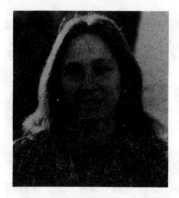

GAIL E. BUTTERFIELD, PH.D.

Assistant Professor and Assistant Nutritionist, Agricultural Experiment Station, Department of Nutritional Sciences, University of California, Berkeley. Author of research reports and publication on biology, anatomy and nutrition. Currently conducting clinical research in energy and nutrient utilization of active people. Member of American College of Sports Medicine and Society for Nutrition Educations. Sigma Xi.

Fat, protein, and carbohydrate are the nutrients known to act as fuels for muscular work. These nutrients are present in varying proportions in all foods, and the mechanism by which they are released from foods to become fuels to the cells is the topic of this paper. To insure a common vocabulary, these nutrient classes will be defined, their non-fuel functions in the body briefly described, and their possible food sources discussed. The steps in the process by which the body then turns these foods into fuels will be presented and recommendations made as to the amounts of each of these nutrients required by athletes.

Fats, or more correctly, lipids, are defined as those elements in food or tissues which are soluable in organic solvents, such as alcohol[1]. In reality, this category of nutrient is very diverse, and consists primarily of triglycerides, phospholipids, and sterols, the most prominent of which is cholesterol.

Triglycerides may be present in food, or synthesized in the liver and intestine, and present the most space-efficient form of energy storage in the body, contributing 9 kilocalories per gram. The triglyceride molecule is composed of a glycerol moiety to which three fatty acids of varying length are attached. It is these fatty acids, long chains of hydrogenated carbon atoms, which provide the fuel for muscular work. Fatty acids may be saturated (containing all the hydrogen atoms possible), or unsaturated (capable of accepting some hydrogen atoms). Linoleic acid is an essential poly-unsaturated fatty acid[2] i.e., necessary for proper function, but not made in the body. Other poly-unsaturated fatty acids are the precursors to the lipid hormones, prostaglandins.

Phospholipids, as a class of lipids, are also present in food or synthesized in the liver and small intestine. They consist of a glycerol moiety bound to two fatty acids, one of which is often linoleic acid, and a third compound which generally contains phosphorus (thus the name "phospholipid") and nitrogen. The phospholipid molecule is capable of interfacing between an aqueous and a lipid phase, and thus becomes, among other things, integral part of cell membranes.

Cholesterol is a complex molecule found in foods and synthesized normally in the liver. It is the common starting point in the synthesis of steroid hormones (testosterone, estrogen, and active Vitamin D being important examples), and is also an integral part of all cell membranes.

Carbohydrates, as a nutrient class, are typified as various groups of hydrated carbon atoms. Simple sugars, such as glucose, and fructose and galactose, upon conversion in the liver, represent the potential fuel forms of carboyhydrate. Other simple sugars, such as ribose and deoxyribose, make up part of the DNA and RNA molecules which control protein synthesis. Sometimes found free in foods, the simple sugars more usually result from the digestion of the more complex naturally occurring entities, disaccarides (double sugars) and polysaccharides, such as starch and glycogen.

Disaccharides, exemplified by sucrose, maltose, and lactose, occur in foods and consist of two simple sugars joined together. The more complex carbohydrates, the starches, glycogen, and fiber, consist of longer chains of these simple forms of carbohydrate. Starch is a general term for polymers of

TABLE 1. Composition of Various Foods, % of Wet Weight

	Animal			Vegetable			
Component	Muscle (beef)	Milk	Eggs	Fruits (apple)	Vegetables (spinach)	Grains (corn)	Beans (dry)
Water	64.7	89	75.5	85.5	95	71.6	23.5
Simple CHO	Trace	4.5	1.2	11.0	2	7.5	2.4
Complex CHO	Trace	None		Trace		14.5	35.2
Fiber	None	None	None	3.7	.6	2.8	17.7
Triglycerides & Phospholipids	18	3.5	10.5	Trace	.3	1.1	5.5
Cholesterol	.3	.07	.5	None	None	None	None
Protein	17	3.2	12	.2	2.1	2.5	10

Derived from values in Briggs and Calloway, Nutrition and Physical Fitness, Saunders, 1979, and USDA Agricultural Handbook #8.

glucose which are the storage form of carbohydrate in plants, whereas glycogen is a somewhat similar molecule produced for carbohydrate storage in animals. Storage of energy as carbohydrate is less space-efficient than storage as fat, glycogen and starch contributing only 4 kilocalories per gram. These polymers are also stored with large quantities of water (3 grams of water per gram of glycogen[3]), which results in further energy dilution.

"Fiber" is a general term for non-digestible complex carbohydrates, and similar substances, such as cellulose, pectin, and lignins, which are produced by plants and which function in the animal body to promote gut motility.

Proteins, as a nutrient class, consists of long chains of the building blocks called amino acids. The element which characterizes proteins is nitrogen, the center of the amino group which gives these blocks their name. Nine of the 22 amino acids known to make up the mammalian body have been found to be essential, that is, necessary for life and not produced in adequate amounts within the body itself[4]. The remaining thirteen forms may be synthesized within the liver and kidney from other amino acids in the diet, provided adequate amino groups are provided. All amino acids must be present at the site of protein synthesis at the time of synthesis in order that any protein may be constructed[5].

The proteins synthesized within the body from the amino acids provided in food act as structural (connective tissue), regulatory (hormones), and catalytic (enzymes) agents, as well as providing the contractile machinary for muscular work.

These individual nutrient classes are found together in all foods, along with other nutrients (such as vitamins, minerals, and water) important to optimal functioning of the organism. The proportion and form of each nutrient found in the various food sources depends upon the source itself. As can be seen in Table 1, animal foods represent the major source of fat in the diet, and the only source of cholesterol. Vegetable foods provide the most significant source of carbohydrate, both simple and complex. However, even within these two classes of foods, there is much variety in the proportion of nutrients provided by any given food (See Table 1), and in the major micro-nutrients which accompany the fuel sources.

Muscle products contain significant amounts of iron, zinc, and vitamin B_6, all nutrients necessary for protein metabolism. Milk and other dairy products represent a major source of calcium, a nutrient necessary for muscle contraction and relaxation, nerve conduction, and maintenance of bone mass. Eggs are a very rich nutrient source, containing everything necessary for the growth of an organism. Fruits, especially citrus fruits, contain, in addition to fuel, significant amounts of ascorbic acid (Vitamin C) and folic acid, necessary, respectively for the integrity of connective tissue and for cell division. Vegetables contain appreciable amounts of the electrolytes, potassium (K), sodium (Na), and magnesium (Mg), and of vitamin A, all nutrients responsible for the maintenance of cellular integrity.

Grains provide the B vitamins, especially riboflavin, thiamin, and niacin, which are essential for the release of energy stored in foods. Beans represent a good source of most nutrients, being an especially good low-fat source of zinc, iron, and the B vitamins[6].

Digestion, the process by which these nutrients in foods are released for use by the cells, is a sequential enzymatic breakdown of the complex molecules to their simpler forms. This process occurs throughout the upper gastro-intestinal tract, in the stomach and small intestine specifically, and is accomplished with the aid of enzymes and other secretions from the gut itself, the pancreas, and the liver. The process is highly controlled to prevent "auto-digestion" of the gut lining. The enzymes are secreted only in response to stimuli—either direct activation of the enzyme-producing cells by specific moieties in the lumen of the gut, or indirect activation via hormones produced elsewhere in the digestive tract and released in response to the presence of specific substances in the vicinity of the hormone-producing cells. The secretion of these enzymes is subsequently halted by a lack of local stimulation, or as a response to inhibitory hormones secreted at other sites in the system[8].

There is also a neural control of secretion (and gut motility) whereby stretch of the digestive tube due to the presence of food causes intra-gut neurons which impinge on secreting cells to fire and to radiate the need for secretion up and down a local segment of gut. Central nervous system involvement via the parasympathetic nerves to the gut (the vagus nerve from the brain, and the sacral parasympathetic plexus) represents the mechanism by which the sight, smell, or thought of food may initiate secretion of digestive enzymes. It is also through this central nervous system connection that anxiety or tension may cause the inappropriate secretion of digestive enzymes.

Once the various nutrients have been released from foods by digestion, they are absorbed through the gut lining cells into the blood, the force for absorption being either active, requiring the use of energy, or passive, the molecules moving along a concentration gradient[7].

As we have seen, foods are composed of all nutrient classes; thus carbohydrate, fat, and protein all enter the system together. However, in the stomach, these different nutrient classes are "parcelled out" by some mechanisms as yet not understood, and released from the stomach for subsequent digestion in the following order: carbohydrate, protein, and then fat[1]. Thus, the details of the digestion and absorption of each nutrient class will be discussed in that order.

Simple sugars which enter the body require no further digestive action, and arrive at the small intestine within minutes of consumption, ready for rapid absorption. Upon entry into the blood, these compounds are carried to the liver, where they will all be converted to glucose, if necessary. This glucose will then either remain in the liver or enter the general circulation, to be carried to other cells in the body. The rapid rise in blood glucose that accompanies the ingestion of simple sugars (and even disaccharides)[9] elicits the secretion of insulin from the pancreas. This hormone causes the cell membranes to become permeable to glucose, and allows its removal from the blood. This general function of insulin to promote fuel storage may be counter-productive in the event that fuel mobilization is needed for strenuous muscular work.

More complex forms of carbohydrate are enzymatically degraded by the action of amylases (starch-breaking enzymes) and disaccharidases secreted from the salivary glands, the gut lining, and the pancreas. The simple sugars that are released are carried immediately to the liver, where their fate is the same as that of any simple sugar. The rate of arrival at the liver of sugars derived from complex carbohydrates is somewhat slower than that of simple sugars ingested directly, and the concommitant rise in blood glucose is less rapid, eliciting a smaller and more gradual insulin response[10].

The fate of glucose is the same, no matter the source. It is either

1) burned as fuel in the liver,

2) stored in the liver or muscle as glycogen, or, once the immediate fuel needs and glycogen storage needs have been met,

3) converted to fat and stored in that form.

Once stored as fat, the carbon chains cannot be reconverted, in any appreciable amount, to glucose.

Protein is the next class of nutrients to leave the stomach. It is actually partially degraded in the stomach by the action of peptidase enzymes and hydrochloric acid. The remnants of this digestive process leave the stomach and are subsequently acted upon by various peptidases from the pancreas and gut lining, enzymes which cleave the peptide bonds between specific pairs of amino acids. Eventually the long chains of amino acids are converted to free amino acids or di- and tri-peptides. These forms are actively absorbed across the lining of the gut, and carried to the liver. The absorbed amino acids are not only derived from the foods eaten, but also from the enzymes used to digest food (enzymes being proteins themselves). The mix of amino acids presented to the liver may thus be different from that present in the food eaten. This recycling mechanism, amounting to as much as 70 gm of endogenous protein secreted, degraded, and reabsorbed per day[11], minimizes the necessity to eat specific quantities of all the essential amino acids at every meal to allow for adequate protein synthesis. Essential amino acids deficient at any one meal may be made up by the essential amino acids released by degradation of the digestive enzymes secreted in response to the meal. However, the intake of essential amino acids must be adequate over the course of 24 hours, so that the essential amino acid pool is not depleted.

The amino acids presented in the liver may be
1) synthesized into proteins, either liver enzymes or plasma proteins;

2) released to the blood for sebsequent use by other cells; or

3) deaminated (the amino group removed) and the resulting carbon skelton converted to glucose or a fat-like substance called ketones.

In the latter case, the fuels thus produced from amino acids will be used as would any other fuel, being either burned, or converted to glycogen or triglycerides for storage. If the amount of amino acids presented to the liver or to the cells exceeds the protein synthetic needs of those sites, the excess amino acids will be deaminated in the liver and converted to fuel.

There is no extensive store of non-functioning protein or amino acids in the body. The consequent nitrogen-containing waste product of this conversion is urea, a substance which is noxious to the body if present in great amounts. Thus urea must be excreted. This excretion is accomplished through the kidneys and requires water, about 50 ml/gm urea nitrogen excreted (1 gm of urea nitrogen is equivalent to that produced from 6.25 gm of protein). Thus, high protein intakes may lead to dehydration if intake exceeds the need of tissues for protein synthesis, and water consumption is not monitored.

Fats, or lipids, are the last nutrient class to leave the stomach, and their digestion and absorption is more complicated, because lipids are not soluble in water and must therefore be made both to be digested and to be transported in the blood. In discussing the digestion of fat, we will concentrate primarily on the breakdown of triglyceride, as that form represents the major fuel source.

The first step in the digestion of lipids requires the emulsification of dietary fat with bile salts secreted from the liver. The action of these caustic substances is to break the large fat droplets into smaller, more easily suspended particles called micells. These particles have a large surface area upon which the fat digesting enzymes (lipases) can act to break the fatty acids from the glycerol moiety of the triglyceride. One, two, or three of the fatty acids may be removed before the molecules are absorbed across the cell membrane. The subsequent fate of the particles depends upon the length of the fatty acid chain.

Short chain fatty acids (chains of 10 carbons or less) pass through the intestinal cell and go to the liver, where they may be burned as fuel, or elongated and made into triglycerides, along with the "extra" simple sugars and amino acid remnants. These liver-generated triglycerides are coated with a protein and phospholipid coat, which makes them soluble in water. These particles, called lipoproteins, are released from the liver and act to transport the fuel to the cells.

Long chain fatty acids cross the cell membrane of the intestinal cells, and are resynthesized into triglycerides within those cells. These triglycerides, and the cholesterol absorbed intact, are also coated with protein and phospholipid to form water-soluble particles called chylomicrons, which move into the lymphatic capillaries underlying the gut lining. The lymphatic system is a circulatory system separate from the general blood-carrying system, and it eventually dumps its non-cellular contents into the general circulation. The fats thus handled initially avoid going through the liver, and present themselves directly to the cells instead.

The lipoproteins from the liver (very low density lipoproteins), and those from the gut (chylomicra), circulate past the cells of the body, and triglycerides and cholesterol are released from those particles by the action of an enzyme in the capillary walls, lipoprotein lipase (LPL)[12]. This enzyme actually degrades the triglyceride again, freeing the fatty acids to enter the cells, to act as a fuel source or to be reconverted to trigylcerides for energy storage. The remnants of the lipoprotein particles thus produced return to the liver for conversion to other lipoprotein forms.

The subsequent intracellular conversions of these nutrients to energy for muscular work will undoubtedly be the topic of other papers in this symposium. It remains only to make use of the information presented to establish some recommendations for intakes of these nutrients. Two pre-event meals for male athletes presented for evaluation by an eastern university coach will be used to illustrate.

Menu 1 contains a high proportion of protein and simple carbohydrate foods. Approximate analysis of the composition of that menu can be found in Table 2. Only 30 grams of the carbohydrate intake are in the form of complex carbohydrate sources, representing only 10% of the total calories. Also summarized in Table 2, contains a high proportion of complex carbohydrate a somewhat lower protein component, and only a small amount of fat. 75 grams of carbohydrate is from complex sources, representing 28% of the total caloric intake.

TABLE 2. Approximate Analysis of Composition of Two Menus*

	Carbohydrate		Protein		Fat	
	gm	% Total Calories	gm	% Total Calories	gm	% Total Calories
Menu 1	89	28.6	98	31.5	55	40.0
Menu 2	119	44.5	68	25.6	35	30.0

*Determined from ADA diabetic exchange list values.

Looking first at the difference in protein intake between the two diets perspective can be attained by realizing that the protein intake recommended by the Food and Nutrition Board of the National Research Council is 0.8 gm protein/kg body weight, or 56 grams of protein for a 70 kg man[13]. In both cases, this single meal fulfills the total 24-hour requirement for protein. It is frequently felt by athletes and their trainers that the protein requirements of the athlete are greater than that of non-athletes, so that perhaps this intake should not be considered excessive.

MENU #1

10 oz.	broiled steak
3 oz.	scrambled eggs
2.5 oz.	green peas
4 oz.	orange juice
2	slices toast with honey
4 oz.	fruit for salad
1	piece fresh fruit
4 oz.	sherbet 5 oz. tea

MENU #2

2	cups	skim milk
6.5	oz.	spaghetti
7	oz.	meatballs and sauce
1/2	cup	green beans
1		piece fresh fruit
1		roll
1	tsp.	margarine
4	oz.	orange juice
1		piece sponge cake
5	oz.	tea with lemon

However, work done in the Department of Nutritional Sciences, University of California, Berkeley, indicates that under the stimulus of increased physical activity, individuals can lay down lean tissue (as measured by retention of nitrogen) with protein intakes as low as 0.57 gm/kg body weight (or 40 gm/day for a 70 kg man), provided energy intake is adequate to cover energy expenditure[14],[15].

In addition, one must remember the body's inability to handle a sudden large influx of amino acids. If these amino acids are not used for protein synthesis, they will be converted to glucose or fat, with the concommitant accumulation of urea, which must be excreted with associated water and electrolyte losses.

An added consequence of such high protein intakes is an increased loss of calcium in the urine[16],[17]. The actual mechanism by which the loss is accomplished is not yet understood[17], but the response appears to be dose-related: the higher the protein intake, the higher the calcium loss. The long-term effect of such losses on bone mass has not yet been determined.

Thus, the high protein intakes of both Menu 1 and Menu 2 have the potential to deplete the athlete's store of vital nutrients, are not necessary for the maintenance of lean tissue, and may actually result in a diminished ability to perform just at a time when optimum performance is desired.

In regard to the large difference in fat intake between the two proposed meals, Menu 1 proposing 55 gm and Menu 2 only 35 gm, researchers have found that the remnants of VLDL and chylomicron degradation are lipoproteins (intermediate density and low density), found to be associated with an increased risk of coronary heart disease[18]. In addition, the complex requirements for digestion inherent in the nature of fats results in a slow movement of the molecules through the process. Total digestion of a heavy fat meal may take as long as 24 hours. Thus, the digestive system may still be busy digesting the high-fat meal at the time when the blood supply would be better utilized feeding exercising muscles.

The final obvious difference between the two proposed pre-event meals is the percentage of calories which are derived from complex carbohydrate sources. Given what we have discussed about the slower rate of appearance at the liver of simple sugars derived from complex carbohydrate sources, it would appear that the composition of the second menu might more optimally promote the slow burning of glucose or its distribution to glycogen stores.

Given these considerations, the recommendations we would make as to the intake of these various nutrient classes are seen in Table 3. The recommendation for protein is greater than that proposed by the National Research Council for moderately active individuals simply because this recommendation fits more closely the intakes found in exercising populations, even in countries where the food supply is marginal[19]. This intake is equivalent to the normal protein intake of most sedantary or moderately active American men. The recommendation for fat reflects the growing body of information relating total fat intake to risk of coronary heart disease, a condition to which physically active adults are not immune.

TABLE 3. Recommendations for the Athlete

Fat	30% of Total Calories
Protein	1-1.5 grams/kg Body Weight
Simple Carbohydrate	15.5% of Total Calories
Complex Carbohydrate	Remainder of Calories to Meet Energy Needs

All recommendations made here are based primarily on the understanding of the physiological process of digestion. The considerations which have led to these recommendations do not even approach the question of what is the optimum fuel for outstanding physical performance.

REFERENCES CITED:

1. Briggs, G.M. and Calloway, D.H., Nutrition and Physical Fitness, 10th ed., W.B. Saunders, Philadelphia, 1979.

2. Burr, G.O., and Burr, M.M., A New Deficiency Disease Produced by the Rigid Exclusion of Fat from the Diet, J. Biol. Chem., 82:345, 1929.

3. Weis-Fogh, T., Metabolism and Weight Economy in Migrating Animals, Particularly Birds and Insects, in G. Blix (Ed.) Nutrition and Physical Activity, p. 84, Almquist and Wiksell, Uppsala, 1967.

4. Kopple, J.D. and Swenseid, M.E., Evidence that Histidine is an Essential Amino Acid in Normal and Chronically Uremic Men, J. Clin. Invest., 55:881, 1975.

5. Goodhart, R.S., and Shils, M.E., Modern Nutrition in Health and Disease, 6th Ed., Lea and Febiger, Philadelphia, 1980.

6. United States Department of Agriculture, Agriculture Handbook #8, Composition of Foods, U.S. Government Printing Office, Washington, D.C., 1963.

7. Ganong, W.F., Review of Medical Physiology, 9th Ed., Lange Medical Publications, Los Altos, California, 1979.

8. Brooks, F.P., Chey, W.Y., Go, V.L.W., Hansky, J., and Konturek, J.J., Second International Conference on Gastrointestinal Hormones, Digestive Diseases and Sciences, 24(6):478, 1979.

9. Crapo, P.A., Reaven, G., and Olefsky, J., Plasma and Insulin Response to Orally Administered Simple and Complex Carbohydrates, Diabetes, 25(9):741, 1976.

10. Coulson, A., Greenfield, M., Kraemer, F., Tobey, T., and Reaven, G., Effect of Source of Dietary Carbohydrates on Plasma Glucose and Insulin Responses to Test Meals in Normal Subjects, Am. J. Clin. Nutr., 33:1279, 1980.

11. Munro, H., Mammalian Protein Metabolism, Vol. 3, New York, Academic Press, 1969, p. 237-262.

12. Korn, E.P., Clearing Factor, a Heparin-Activated Lipoprotein Lipase. II. Substrate Specificity and Activation of Coconut Oil, J. Biol. Chem., 215:15, 1955.

13. National Research Council, Recommended Daily Allowances, 9th Ed., Washington, D.C., National Academy of Sciences, 1980.

14. Butterfield-Hodgdon, G., and Calloway, D.H., Protein Utilization in Men Under Two Conditions of Energy Balance and Work, Fed. Proc., 39:377, 1977 (Abstract)

15. Butterfield, G., and Calloway, D.H., Protein Utilization in Men Fed Inadequate Energy at Three Levels of Work, Fed. Proc., 1981 (Abstract)

16. Margen, S., Chu, J-J, Kaufmann, N.A., and Calloway, D.G., Studies in Calcium Metabolism, I. The Calciuretic Effect of Dietary Protein, Am. J. Clin. Nutr., 27:584, 1974.

17. Allen, L.H., Block, G.D., Wood, R.J., and Bryce, G.F., The Role of Insulin and Parathyroid Hormone in the Protein-Induced Calciuria of Man, Nutr. Res., 1:3, 1981.

18. Kannel, W.B., Castelli, W.P., Gordon, R., and McNamara, P.M., Serum Cholesterol, Lipoproteins, and the Risk of Coronary Heart Disease. The Framingham Study, Ann. Internal Med., 74:1. 1971.

19. Rand, W.M., Uauy, R., and Scrimshaw, N.S., eds., Protein-Energy Requirements in Developing Countries: Results of Internationally Coordinated Research, Report of a Workshop of the International Union of Nutritional Sciences, August, 1981, University of California, Berkeley.

Fats and Carbohydrates as Determinants of Athletic Performance

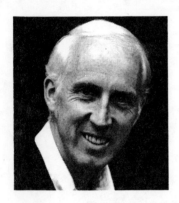

DAVID L. COSTILL, PH.D.

Director of Human Performance Laboratory and Professor, Departments of Physical Education and Biology, Ball State University, Muncie, Indiana. Leading educator and researcher in the areas of physical and sports medicine. Has published over 125 articles, participated in symposia and workshops worldwide, and past president of American College of Sports Medicine.

It is generally agreed that the availability of endogenous fuels plays a critical role during athletic performance. Specifically, research on carbohydrate metabolism has shown that when the glycogen stores in exercised muscles are exhausted, the muscles are unable to continue high intensity activity[19],[24]. Although fats also serve as a critical fuel during activity of long duration, it is the glycogen in muscle and the glucose in blood that are the primary sources of energy for most althetic events. The intensity of most athletic events demands that the most readily available and combustible fuel (carbohydrate) be used to produce the energy for muscle contraction. Unfortunately, the storage of this energy source (glycogen) is sometimes less than that needed for optimal performance. Consequently, dietary regimens have been proposed to maximize the athlete's carbohydrate stores and to minimize the rate of their depletion during training and competition[3].

FUELS FOR EXERCISE

Since the early studies of Christensen and Hansen[7], it has been generally agreed that both lipids and carbohydrates contribute to energy metabolism during endurance exercise. Although proteins are important as the building blocks of the body, there is limited evidence to suggest that they provide a major energy source for muscle. The fraction of energy derived from carbohydrates during prolonged exercise is dependent on a number of factors, including the exercise intensity, the physical condition of the athlete, the mode of exercise, environmental temperature, and the intake of carbohydrates before and during the activity.

First, let us consider the type of substrates used during athletic events involving explosive, short term (less than 15-20 minutes) muscular activity. Sprint runners, swimmers and others who must exert near maximal muscle force, obtain nearly 100% of their energy from muscle glycogen. In these events the flow of oxygen to the working muscles does not adequately meet the demands for oxidative metabolism, thereby requiring that most of the enrgy (ATP) for muscle contraction be generated via glycogenolysis, the anaerobic breakdown of glycogen. Saltin and Karlsson[25] have shown that the rate of muscle glycogen utilization is exponentially related to exercise intensity. While very little muscle glycogen is combusted (about 0.3 mmol/kg x min-l) during exercise such as walking (10 to 20% of one's aerobic capacity), Hultman[20] has reported a maximum rate of glycogen usage of nearly 40 mmol/kg x min-l during maximal isometric contractions.

Thus, in events that impose repeated, near maximal bursts of effort, muscle glycogen reserves can be drastically diminished. Even in sports like football, soccer and basketball, intense training and competition will tend to lower the muscle glycogen stores, thereby limiting the athlete's ability to perform at an optimal level.

In long-term exercise, longer than 20-30 min, not all of the ATP produced is from the endogenous sugar stores. Though lipids contribute substantially to the energy pool in events like the marathon, still it is muscle glycogen and blood glucose that serve as the critical fuel source for repeated muscle contractions. During the early minutes of exercise, before the oxygen transport system has fully compensated for the sudden increase in exercise metabolism, muscle glycogen is used at a greater rate than during the latter stages of effort[5]. Concomitantly, lipids contribute little to the energy pool at the beginning of an endurance exercise session, but may be the largest contributor in the final minutes of the activity.

Aside from the duration and intensity of exercise, there are other factors that influence the muscle's choice of fuels. Fink, et al.[16] have noted that muscle glycogen depletion is accelerated (+76%) during exercise in the heat (temp. = 41° C, R.H. = 55%) as compared to similar activity in a cold environment (temp. = 9° C, R.H. = 55%). Even the training status of the athlete will have a bearing on the muscle's choice of substrates for energy. As a consequence of endurance training, the oxygen supply to working muscles is improved and the tissue's capacity to conduct oxidative metabolism is enhanced. Consequently, the endurance trained muscle demonstrates a greater capacity to oxidize fats and thereby spare the use of glycogen. This shift in substrate utilization constitutes one of the most critical adaptations for the endurance athlete, for it is one mechanism that has a direct influence on performance in events that are limited by a lack of stored carbohydrates (i.e. glycogen).

It is well known that diet before and during exercise can have an influence on the muscle's choice of fuels. Early studies by Christensen and Hansen[7] demonstrated that individuals who were fed diets rich in carbohydrates tended to derive a large fraction of their energy from carbohydrates during steady-state exercise. More recently, we have noted that ingesting a sugar solution in the 60 minutes before exercise produced a marked rise in blood glucose, insulin and carbohydrate metabolism during submaximal treadmill running. Even when our subjects were given sugar solutions after the start of exercise, the amount of carbohydrate oxidized was significantly greater than when they were given only water. It should be noted here that the intake of a glucose or sucrose solution in the final minutes (30-60 min) before exercise often resulted in a rapid decrease in blood glucose when the subjects started to exercise[11]. In some cases we observed that the participants were hypoglycemic (less than 50 mg/100 ml) after only 10 min of exercise. Despite having a lower blood sugar level the subjects continued to combust a large quantity of carbohydrates, principally muscle glycogen.

Based on muscle biopsy studies, we concluded that the intake of sugar solutions before exercise resulted in a series of events that might negatively influence endurance performance. The sugar drink elevated the subjects' blood glucose and insulin, which induced a rapid removal of glucose by the muscle when activated to contract. Under these conditions the uptake of glucose appears to be more rapid than the liver or intestinal ability to supply glucose to the blood. Consequently, blood glucose declines and the muscle fibers must rely more heavily on their glycogen stores for fuel. This greater use of muscle glycogen depletes the muscle's supply, which eventually results in exhaustion for the endurance athlete.

But, what athletes need to worry about this problem? Cyclists, marathon runners and long distance swimmers are the athletes who must be concerned with depletion of muscle glycogen, and who might suffer the negative effects of ill-timed sugar feedings.

In our first studies on muscle glycogen depletion with distance runners we were surprised to find that at exhaustion, there was still a reasonable amount of glycogen remaining in the thigh (vastus lateralis) and calf (gastrocnemius) muscles[14]. This was in contrast with the almost complete emptying of glycogen from the thigh muscles seen in exhausted cyclists[22]. These findings led us to assume that the determining factor for exhaustion was different for these two forms of exercise. In cycling it is possible to continue the exercise even when the muscles are quite fatigued, but at a reduced cadence and force on the pedals. Runners, on the other hand, cannot continue beyond the fatigue point where the muscles' tension capabilities might risk literal collapse.

The point here is that the degree of glycogen depletion at various stages of fatigue and exhaustion may vary depending on the mode of exercise. Swimmers, for example, empty their arm muscle glycogen during each daily training session (unpublished).

It should be noted that the demands placed on muscle glycogen are not shared equally by all the fibers in an exercising muscle. It has been shown that during prolonged exercise at less than 70 to 80% of the subject's aerobic capacity (V°_2 max), glycogen depletion is greatest in the endurance type fibers (Slow Twitch or Type I), which suggests that these fibers are given the greatest responsibility for tension development at this level of effort[13],[17]. As the intensity of exercise increases toward or above the V°_2 max level, the Slow Twitch fibers are joined by the more anaerobic type fibers (Fast Twitch or Type II), to produce greater tension and speed. Thus, the intensity of exercise has a bearing on the selective depletion of glycogen and graded exhaustion in specific muscle fibers. This means that the pool of muscle fibers available for meeting the demands of the exercise task will gradually be diminished in long term activity, and the sensation of effort will be increased.

This information has direct application to athletic training and competition. Training sessions that emphasize intense bursts or sprints (intervals) will result in a large breakdown of muscle glycogen in both Slow and Fast Twitch fibers, which might be more costly to the athlete than a training bout of long steady activity (e.g. distance running). On a day-to-day basis, training of this type will leave the athlete with less than optimal levels of glycogen in the fibers that are needed for maximal performance and heavy training. As a result, the athlete may experience the sluggish sensation of being "overtrained."

Blood-borne glucose is the other major contributor to the carbohydrate needs of the muscle. At rest the uptake of glucose accounts for less than 10% of the total oxygen consumption by muscle[2]. During moderate to strenuous bicycle exercise, however, the net glucose uptake by the leg muscles increases 10 to 20-fold above the resting value[27]. As the time of exercise is extended, the fraction of energy derived from blood glucose increases and may account for 75 to 90% of the muscle's carbohydrate needs[27]. This taxation on the blood glucose pool demands that the liver keep pace by increasing its output of glucose to prevent hypoglycemia (low blood sugar). Consequently, the liver must break down its glycogen reserves or produce glucose from other precursors, such as alanine and branch chained amino acids.

Unfortunately, the human liver has a limited glycogen supply and is not always capable of producing enough glucose to keep pace with the muscle's expectations, though in endurance-trained, well-fed athletes this is not a problem. In these individuals there is substantial use of fats as fuel, and their carbohydrate stores are large enough to tolerate several hours of heavy exercise without becoming hypoglycemic. Untrained, poorly fed individuals, on the other hand, will show a gradual decline in blood glucose during endurance exercise lasting 1-2 hours. Thus, it seems low blood glucose in a problem for athletes that are exercising for long periods, but not for those engaged in short, intense effort. To the contrary, in events like sprint swimming and running, blood glucose is usually quite elevated after the event, as a result of the hormonal stimulation to release large quantities of glucose from the liver.

There is, of course, one option for those who risk exertional hypoglycemia. Fluids containing carbohydrates can be ingested during the exercise to supplement the liver's carbohydrate stores. Recent studies, however, have shown that carbohydrate intake during exercise does not improve the total work output in 120 min. of exhaustive exercise[21]. In that study, the subjects were highly trained cyclists who did not show signs of hypoglycemia during the control treatment (no carbohydrate feedings). We did, however, note that the sugar drinks did increase the total work output during the final 30 minutes of the exercise.

As mentioned earlier, one of the major adaptations to endurance training is the accommodation for fat metabolism. Based on our laboratory measurements of respiratory gas exchange (carbon dioxide and oxygen), we have noted that trained distance runners occasionally derive as much as 75% of their energy from fat during 60 minutes of treadmill running at about 70% of $V°_2$ max[12].

At this point it should be made clear that the fats oxidized by muscles to form ATP are not the same as those stored inside the fat cell or inside the muscle. The storage form of fat is triglyceride, a complex of glycerol and free fatty acids (FFA). It is the FFA that enter into the process of metabolism, but this requires the breakdown of triglycerides to make the less complex FFA available for entry into the muscle fibers. This mobilization of FFA is accomplished with the aid of special enzymes that are hormonally activated.

At the onset of exercise, FFA are in limited supply but still contribute to the energy needs of the muscle. Since the process involved in the mobilization of these important lipids is slow to get started, the individual may exercise for 30-40 min. before the rate of mobilization of FFA equals or exceeds the rate of utilization in the exercising fibers.

The rate of FFA utilization is controlled, in part, by its concentration in blood[18]. The increased mobilization of FFA from adipose tissue elevates plasma FFA, which subsequently increases the rate of its oxidation in the working muscle. Since FFA serve as an alternate to carbohydrates for muscular energy, their increased availability tends to spare the use of muscle glycogen and, thereby, improves endurance performance[9,10].

In addition to the FFA from the adipose tissue triglyceride, a portion of the fats oxidized during prolonged exercise are derived from the hydrolysis (breakdown) of blood and intramuscular triglycerides[13],[15]. Though the contribution of plasma triglyceride to the muscle's energy needs is relatively small, intramuscular lipid stores have been shown to decrease 30% and 50% during 30 and 100 km races, respectively[13],[15].

Due to the intense nature of most athletic events, lipids contribute much less to the muscle energy needs than do carbohydrates. Only in events that are limited by glycogen depletion will enhanced FFA oxidation serve to improve performance.

Thus, it is apparent that optimal endurance sports performance is strongly influenced by the availability of both carbohydrates (glycogen and glucose) and fats (FFA). It is generally agreed that nutrition plays a central role in both storage and utilization of these fuels. There is little doubt that one must emphasize carbohydrates in the diet since their storage in liver and muscle is limited. Fats, on the other hand, are stored in abundance and need only be mobilized for use.

DIETARY NEEDS OF THE ATHLETE

The untrained, human skeletal muscle generally stores 80-100 mmol glucose units/kg of tissue despite a diet high in carbohydrates. The leg muscles of trained distance runners, on the other hand, often contain 150-250 mmol/kg after two days of rest and a mixed diet containing 350-450 grams of carbohydrate. This large storage of muscle glycogen is a biological adaptation to accommodate the daily usage. This appears to be a factor related to chronic exercise (training) rather than the effects of an acute bout of exercise. That is to say, an untrained subject cannot hope to increase his/her glycogen stores simply by exercising hard and then eating a diet rich in carbohydrates.

The rate of muscle glycogen resynthesis following exhaustive exercise appears to be related to the activity of a special muscle enzyme (glycogen synthetase), and the carbohydrate content of the subject's diet[3,23]. Exercise depletion of muscle glycogen results in a marked elevation in this enzyme, which facilitates the storage of glycogen when accompanied by a rich carbohydrate diet.

During repeated days of heavy endurance training we have noted that muscle glycogen resynthesis is very small when subjects ate a mixed diet containing 300-350 grams/day[8]. Consequently, after several days of this diet-exercise regimen the athletes tended to have very low leg muscle glycogen values (15-20 mmol/kg tissue) and were unable to perform even moderately heavy exercise. When the same subjects were fed a high carbohydrate diet (600 grams/day), the daily, pre-exercise muscle glycogen values remained above 100 mmol/kg and the subjects perceived the daily exercise as much less difficult. Thus, it appears that athletes who train exhaustively on successive days must consume a diet rich in carbohydrates if they wish to minimize the threat of chronic exhaustion often associated with the accumulated depletion of muscle glycogen.

It appears, therefore, that the composition of the athlete's diet may be critical to her/his glycogen reserves. A logical question might be, "what type carbohydrates are best?" or "are there differences in the different carbohydrates with regard to their storage in muscle?" Although we have examined this question, in part, by testing the storage of glycogen following the intake of complex (starch) and simple (glucose) carbohydrates, the entire answer must wait further study. Since there are different hormone responses associated with several of the carbohydrate molecules (e.g., dextrins and fructose), it is possible that there may be some difference in their impact on glycogen synthesis.

It is apparent, therefore, that different diets can markedly influence muscle glycogen stores, and that the higher the glycogen content the better is one's potential for endurance performance. Studies by Bergstrom and associates[1,4,6] demonstrated that exercise manipulation could elevate muscle glycogen stores to very high levels (above 200 mmol/kg).

It was proposed that the optimal plan to achieve "maximal" glycogen storage (often termed glycogen loading or glycogen super compensation) in preparation for endurance competition, should involve an exhaustive training bout about one week before competition. For the following 3 days the athlete's diet should be almost entirely fat and protein, thus keeping the glycogen depots very low and possibly elevating glycogen to high levels. Thereafter, the athlete should consume a rich carbohydrate diet for the days leading up to competition. While this regimen has been shown to produce very large muscle glycogen stores, it does cause a great deal of discomfort for the athlete during the high fat-protein segment of the regimen.

Recently, we have conducted studies to compare the above "glycogen loading" protocol to a dietary regimen that allowed the subjects to eat a normal mixed diet (50% of Calories from carbohydrates) in place of the high fat-protein portion of the classical routine[26]. We found no difference between the two regimens and have concluded that the athlete can insure a very large muscle glycogen storage simply by eating a carbohydrate rich diet in the 48-72 hours before the endurance event, provided he/she rests during that period.

We also noted that such efforts to superload the muscle with glycogen has little or no influence on performance in events lasting less than 90 minutes. Subsequent studies from our laboratory have, however, demonstrated that such dietary manipulation is critical to participants in events lasting longer than this (e.g., marathon).

CONCLUSION

Since the endogenous stores of carbohydrates are limited, it is understandable that the use of an alternate fuel source, such as fat, could serve to spare muscle and liver glycogen, thereby improving performance in endurance events. Though we have demonstrated this fact experimentally by injecting heparin, thereby elevating FFA, there are few dietary ways to accomplish the same feat[9].

Some drugs, namely caffeine, have been found to promote fat oxidation and improve performance in long lasting, exhaustive events[10,21]. When administered 60 minutes before exercise, caffeine stimulated an increase in fat metabolism and a decline in muscle glycogen usage. It was also noted that caffeine ingestion (4 to 5 mg/kg body wt.) produced a lessening of the subjective rating of effort. Thus, we concluded that at least part of the performance advantage associated with the ingestion of caffeine was psychological in nature. Despite the endurance advantage provided by the ingestion of dietary items like coffee and tea, the ethical use of these drinks must be considered in light of their stimulating effects of the sympathetic nervous system.

Based on the preceding discussion, it should be obvious that the body's carbohydrate and fat stores play an important role in maximal athletic performance. More importantly, the interaction between these two fuels is critical to endurance athletes, who must rely on lipid metabolism as an alternate energy source in an effort to spare their limited muscle and liver glycogen supply.

REFERENCES

1. Ahlborg, B.J., et al. Human muscle glycogen content and capacity for prolonged exercise after different diets. **Foersvarsmedicin** 3: 85-99, 1967.

2. Anres, R., et al. The quantitatively minor role of carbohydrate in oxidative metabolism by skeletal muscle in intact man in the basal state. Measurements of oxygen and glucose uptake and carbon dioxide and lactate production in the forearm. **J.Clin.Invest.** 35:671-682, 1956.

3. Astrand, P.O. Nutrition and athletic performance. **Fed. Proced.** 26:1772-1777, 1967.

4. Bergstrom, J., et al., Diet, muscle glycogen and physical performance. **Acta Physiol Scand.** 71:140-150, 1967.

5. Bergstrom, J. and E. Hultman. The effect of exercise on muscle glycogen and electrolytes in normals. **Scand J Clin Lab Invest,** 18:16-20, 1966.

6. Bergstrom, J. and E. Hultman. Muscle glycogen synthesis after exercise: An enhancing factor localized to the muscle cells in man. **Nature.** 210: 309-310, 1966.

7. Christensen, E.H. and O. Hansen III. Arbeitsfahigkeit Ernahrung. **Skand Arch Physiol.,** 81:160-171, 1939.

8. Costill, D.L., et al., Muscle glycogen utilization during prolonged exercise on successive days. **J.Appl.Physiol.,** 31:834-838, 1971.

9. Costill, D.L., et al., Effects of elevated plasma FFA and insulin on muscle glycogen usage during exercise. **J.Appl.Physiol.,** 43:695-699, 1977.

10. Costill, D.L., et al., Effects of caffeine ingestion on metabolism and exercise performance. **Med Sci Sports,** 10:155-158, 1978.

11. Costill, D.L., et al., The role of dietary carbohydrates in muscle glycogen resynthesis following strenuous running. **Am.J.Clin.Nut.,** (In Press).

12. Costill, D.L., et al., Lipid metabolism in skeletal muscle of endurance trained males and females. **J.Appl.Physiol.,** 47:787-791, 1979.

13. Costill, D.L., et al., Glycogen depletion pattern in human muscle fibers during distance running. **Acta Physiol Scand.,** 89:374-383, 1973.

14. Costill, D.L., et al., Muscle glycogen utilization during exhaustive running. **J.Appl.Physiol.,** 31:353-356, 1971.

15. Essen, B. Intramuscular substrate utilization during prolonged exercise. **Ann N Y Acad Sci.,** 301:30-44, 1977.

16. Fink, W.J., et al., Leg muscle metabolism during exercise in the heat and cold. **Europ J Appl Physiol.,** 34:183-190, 1975.

17. Gollnick, P.D., et al., Glycogen depletion patterns in human skeletal muscle fibers during prolonged work. **Pfluegers Arch.,** 344:1-12, 1973.

18. Havel, R.J., et al., Uptake and release of free fatty acids and other metabolism in the legs of exercising man. **J.Appl.Physiol.,** 23:90-96, 1966.

19. Hultman, E., Studies on muscle metabolism of glycogen and active phosphate in man with special reference to exercise and diet. **Scand J Clin Lab Invest,** 94:1-64 (suppl.), 1967.

20. Hultman, E., Muscle fuel for competition. **Physician Sports Med,** January 1979.

21. Ivy, J.L., et al., Influence of caffeine and carbohydrate feedings on endurance performance. **Med Sci Sports,** 11:6-11, 1979.

22. Pernow, B. and B. Saltin, Availability of substrates and capacity for prolonged heavy exercise in man. **J.Appl.Physiol.,** 31:416-422, 1971.

23. Piehl, K., Time course for refilling of glycogen stores in human muscle fibers following exercise-induced glycogen depletion. **Acta Physiol Scand,** 90:297-302, 1974.

24. Saltin, B. and L. Hermansen. Glycogen stores and prolonged severe exercise. In: Blix G., ed. **Nutrition and Physical Activity.** Sweden: Almquist and Wiksell, 5:32-46, 1967.

25. Saltin, B. and J. Karlsson. Muscle glycogen utilization during work of different intensities. In: Pernow, B. and B. Saltin (ed): **Muscle Metabolism during Exercise.** New York, Plenum Press, 1971.

26. Sherman, W.M., et al., The effect of exercise-diet manipulation on muscle glycogen and its subsequent utilization during performance. **Int.J.Sports Med.** (In Press).

27. Wahren, J., et al., Glucose metabolism during exercise in man. **J. Clin.Invest.** 50: 2715-2725, 1971.

Summary

Dr. Butterfield opened this session by reviewing the sources and basic structure of dietary fats, proteins, and carbohydrates and how they are assimilated by the body. The fate of these nutrients once digested and the primary functions they serve was discussed. Examples of how the relative caloric contribution of these substrates can be modified for enhancement of health and performance were presented.

Dr. Costill reviewed the scientific basis of dietary intake and endurance training regimens that enhance and conserve muscle glycogen stores. He provided the rationale for carbohydrate stores being the limiting factor for strenuous endurance type exercise exceeding 90 minutes. He also discussed the role of blood-borne and muscle free fatty acids as metabolic substrates during exercise.

Of interest to the participants was the use of coffee to enhance endurance performance, a concept also presented by Dr. Costill. That the release of free fatty acids into the blood by the caffeine in coffee can enhance endurance performance has been demonstrated in the laboratory, but not under race conditions. Some people (estimated to be 20%) do not respond and tend to feel worse, with nausea and headaches. The amount of coffee used should be adjusted for body weight; 4-5 milligrams of caffeine per kilogram of body weight appears sufficient and needs to be consumed approximately one hour prior to the event. Only performances requiring continuous activity of 90 minutes or longer will probably be influenced. Reference was made to evidence of possible association of caffeine with such disorders as ulcers, cancer, heart disease and birth defects. Also, the diuretic effects of coffee and tea were discussed, with recommendations that they should be avoided when retention of body fluids is critical.

The popularization by Dr. George Sheehan of the use of beer as a fluid replacement following exercise was brought to the speakers, attention for comments. The general consensus was that beer is not a good fluid replacement during or following exercise for the following reasons:

(1) it is slow to leave the stomach due to its relatively high osmolalilty;

(2) the alcohol in beer produces a diuresis and aggrevates dehydration; and

(3) alcohol requires energy to be metabolized by the liver. These potential detrimental characteristics of alcohol mitigate against the routine use of beer for fluid replacement, although no direct evidence of detrimental consequences has been reported.

Dr. Costill referred to evidence supporting the idea that all forms of carbohydrates are equally effective in replenishing muscle glycogen stores depleted by vigorous exercise. Super compensation is achieved in highly-trained athletes if 8 grams of carbohydrate per kilogram of body weight are consumed over a 48-hour period, during which time no strenuous activity is performed. Super compensation generally appears helpful in endurance events exceeding 90 minutes of continuous exercise.

Also, the possibility that glycogen depletion of specific muscle fibers occurs in activities of total shorter duration needs to be considered. However, any athlete performing vigorous endurance exercise during daily training sessions should maintain a relatively high carbohydrate intake.

Not much is known about the fate of various forms of carbohydrate consumed during vigorous endurance exercise. For events of short duration carbohydrate intake has no effect, whereas performance of endurance events approaching two hours or longer can be enhanced by the replenishing of muscle, liver or blood carbohydrate stores.

It was re-emphasized that one of the major results of endurance training is an enhanced ability to mobilize and oxidize free fatty acids during exercise. This can be a realistic goal of long training runs; shorter bouts of high-intensity exercise do not produce this effect.

Dr. Butterfield discussed with several participants the effects of exercise on protein requirements. It appears that low or moderate intensity exercise does not increase the body's need for protein, whereas longer, endurance-type exercise may increase specific amino acid utilization. However, the intake of protein by most athletes is so high that there is no general real risk of a protein deficiency, even where exercise may increase protein use.

FLUID INTAKE AND ATHLETIC PERFORMANCE

The Body's Need for Fluids

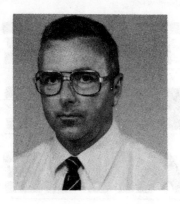

JOHN E. GREENLEAF, PH.D.

Research Physiologist, Life Sciences Directorate, NASA Ames Research Center. Recognized expert on the effects of heat, exercise, bedrest and dehydration upon human physical perfomance. Has published 150 scientific articles, and served as editor of International Journal of Biometeorology and Journal of Applied Physiology.

Body Fluids During Exercise. The ability of an organism to maintain the relative constancy of the volume and constituents of the "milieu interne," or internal environment, a concept first formulated by the French physiologist Claude Bernard[1], is a basic requisite for survival. Walter Cannon of Harvard University called it homeostasis[2]. The main element of the milieu interne is the extracellular fluid volume (interstitial and plasma volumes) which comprises all body fluids outside the cells (Figure 1).

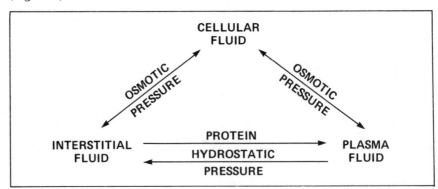

FIGURE 1. Cellular and extracellular fluid compartments: volumes and fractions of body weight.

When body metabolism is increased by physical exercise, numerous constituents in the cellular and extracellular fluids are displaced from their at-rest, or normal concentrations. As a result, various physiological systems are activated that tend to restore these displaced constituents to within their normal limits. Fatigue occurs because of the delay in the restoration process. The phenomenon of fatigue is generally familiar, but its physiological mechanisms remain an enigma. Fatigue results in part from deficits of oxygen, water, or calories that can occur singly or in combination. Under optimal conditions the human body can survive about 10 min without oxygen, 18 days without water, but nearly 60 days without food. In many instances it appears that the body's requirement for these three elements for combating fatigue is in about the same proportion as its respective survival times without them.

When consideration is given to the effect of fluid balance on human performance and fatigue, an inseparable component is the control of body temperature. Physical exercise raises core temperature in direct proportion to the load imposed, and dehydration results in an additional increment in temperature[8]. When compared with the day-to-day variability of many physical and chemical parameters in the body, the smallest variability was found in body temperature, plasma sodium, chloride, and osmolality[22]. This suggests these parameters are of major importance for optimal physiological function. Thus, a complete discussion of the effects of exercise and fluid balance must also consider thermoregulation[7].

In this paper I will discuss the anatomy of body fluid distribution and exchange, and the interaction between body fluids, sweating, and thermoregulation.

ANATOMY OF BODY FLUID DISTRIBUTION AND EXCHANGE

In normal, healthy people total body water comprises 50% to 70% of the body weight. The higher the percentage of body fat the lower the percentage of water because fat contains less water than muscle (Table 1). The average body water content in the general population is about 61% of the body weight[19]. Turnover of body water requires 11-13 days[23]; the total volume is regulated daily to within±0.22% (±150 g) of the body weight[28], and plasma volume to within ±0.7% (±25g)[9]. A typical water balance in a normal, resting person is given in Table 2. With exercise, the values for sweating and water intake would be increased. Under stressful conditions, voluntary fluid intake lags behind water loss, a condition termed involuntary dehydration[12].

TABLE 1. Weight and water content of body tissue from a 70.6 kg man.*

Tissue	Percent of body weight	Percent water content
Striated muscle	31.6	79.5
Skeleton	14.8	31.8
Adipose tissue	13.6	50.1
Skin	7.8	64.7
Lungs	4.2	83.7
Liver	3.4	71.5
Brain and spinal cord	2.5	73.3
Alimentary tract	2.1	79.1
Alimentary tract contents	0.8	—
Heart	0.7	73.7
Kidneys	0.5	79.5
Spleen	0.2	78.7
Pancreas	0.2	73.1
Bile	0.2	—
Teeth	0.1	5.0
Hair	0.1	—
Remaining Tissues		
Liquid	3.7	93.3
Solid	13.5	70.4
Total Body	100.0	67.2

*Modified from ref. 19.

TABLE 2. Typical daily water balance in a resting 70 kg person

Source	Weight, grams	Percent of total
Input:		
Beverage	1200	48
Food Moisture	1000	40
Oxidation within tissues	250	10
Preformed in food	50	2
Total input	2500	100
Output:		
Urine water	1400	56
Skin ⎫	600	24
⎬ insensible water		
Lungs ⎭	300	12
Fecal water	200	8
Sweat	0	0
Total output	2500	100
Water balance (input-output)	0	

Copious water drinking in healthy people is not harmful. Voluntary water intake up to 9,570 ml per day does not alter serum osmolality significantly[16]. The kidneys are the major organs for regulating fluid volume and solute concentration, and with a normally functioning antidiuretic hormone system, they are capable of regulating massive volumes of water. If body water is depleted, the kidneys will concentrate the urine to about 1,400 mOsm/kg and continue to do so until they fail or until water is ingested. Normal kidney function reabsorbs 99% of the 150 liters of glomerular filtrate formed per day; the remaining 1-2 liters are excreted as urine. In pathological conditions large volumes of fluid may be lost daily in various ways: sweating (10-15 liters); diarrhea (5 liters); vomiting (5 liters); and hyperventilation (1-2 liters). With diabetes insipidus, where function of the antidiuretic hormone is impaired, daily urine volume can be 30 liters or more with a corresponding volume of fluid intake.Chronic retention of excess water, owing to excessive secretion of antidiuretic hormone, may result in water intoxication which can be fatal.

Water lost by the body, except through the lungs, is always accompanied by electrolytes, mainly sodium and chloride. The normal constituent composition of the fluid spaces in man is given in Table 3. Sodium is the major cation and chloride the major anion in the extracellular fluid. Changes in plasma sodium concentration indicate, approximately, changes in extracellular fluid volume. Potassium is the principal intracellular cation, and phosphates and protein the major anions. Even though there is a significant difference between the intracellular cation and anion osmolality (175 and 135 = 310 mOsm/kg), the total intracellular osmolality is exactly equal to the total extracellular osmolality (155 and 155 = 310 mOsm/kg). Therefore, essentially equal osmotic concentrations are maintained between two complex fluids of widely different ionic content (Table 3).

TABLE 3. Normal composition of fluid spaces in man.

Fluid space	Cations				Anions			
	Na$^+$	K$^+$	Other$^+$ Ca + Mg	Osmols$^+$	Cl$^-$	HCO^{-3}	Other$^-$ (PO$_4$ + PRO)	Osmols$^-$
	mEq/z	mEq/z	mEq/z	mOsm/kg	mEq/z	mEq/z	mEq/z	mOsm/kg
Extracellular	142	5	8	155	103	27	25	155
Cellular	10	145	20	175	2	8	190	135
Total	152	150	28	330	105	35	215	290

The fluid composition of the body is maintained according to the laws of osmotic pressure:

1. osmotic equilibrium exists between cells and water;

2. nine tenths of the osmotic pressure of the body is maintained by electrolytes, and the remainder by proteins and other macromolecules;

3. water distribution is determined mainly by sodium and potassium distribution;

4. osmotic equilibrium between plasma and red blood cells is achieved mainly by the transfer of water;

5. marked changes in total body water distribution occur, even when the volume of water remains unchanged[4].

INTERACTION BETWEEN FLUIDS, SWEATING, AND THERMOREGULATION

Of the homeothermic mammals, man is unique because of his relatively large potential capacity for heat dissipation by evaporation of sweat. It is mainly this large sweating capacity that allows man to perform high-intensity physical exercise for prolonged periods of time. Without it, the induced hyperthermia would result in heat exhaustion, and perhaps heat stroke and death. Fortunately, in many cases, fatigue and syncope intervene to stop the exertion before heat stroke occurs. Except in unusual evnironmental conditions, the other avenues for heat dissipation (conduction, convection, and radiation) are not as efficient as evaporation for removing heat from the body (because of the high latent heat of water). In a temperate environment, with moderate solar radiation, the primary source of heat is the body's metabolism. Maximal physical exertion for a few minutes can increase the metabolic rate to about 1,800 kcal/hr, about 30 times the basal metabolic rate. If the average "normal" core temperature is 37.0°C (98.6°F), death can occur if the temperature drops to 27.0°C (80.6°F); on the other hand, an increase to only 42.0°C (107.6°F) can also cause death. Thus, overheating appears to be more critical for survival than overcooling. Men have survived with core temperatures between 24.0°C (75.2°F) and 45.6°C (114.1°F)[5]. The lower limit of core termperature for the onset of heat stroke is about 41.5°C (106.8°F), but cases of classical heat stroke have been reported with core temperatures of 40.6°C (105.2°F)[18]. Unacclimated young men, resting in a hot [42°C (107.6°F)] and humid (90% relative humidity) environment, are near their limits of tolerance and consciousness with rectal temperatures of only 38.5°C (101.3°F)[3]. On the other hand, rectal temperatures of 40.0°C-41.1°C (104.1°F-106.1°F) have been reported in runners after a marathon race, without causing ill effects[21]. Although part of the ability to perform high-intensity and long-duration physical exercise is inherited, there is ample evidence that tolerance for higher core temperature and associated enhanced maximal sweating capacity (heat acclimation) can be induced by physical exercise training in a hot environment[24].

Sweat is derived from interstitial fluid. The volume of interstitial fluid is maintained by the transfer of plasma and cellular fluid (Figure 1). Sweating during heat exposure without exercise depletes mainly the extracellular fluid compartment, and sweating during exercise depletes both the extracellular and cellular fluid compartments[17].

One important mechanism—the first line of defense—for maintenance of the interstitial fluid volume during exercise is the shift of plasma to the interstitial space in proportion to the increase in systolic blood pressure, which is directly proportional to exercise intensity[10]. This fluid shift occurs during the first 10 min of exercise and the magnitude of the shift increases from about 6% (180 ml) with moderate exercise[12] to about 16% (500 ml) during peak (maximal) exercise (Figure 2; Table 4). A second and more slowly acting mechanism is the production of water liberated from the metabolism of glycogen during exercise. Oxidation of 500 g of muscle glycogen over a period of 4-6 h could produce 1,500 ml of water[11].

Because continued sweating during prolonged exercise can reach a rate of 800-1,000 ml/h, it is obvious that additional fluid must be provided by drinking. The rise in rectal temperature during exercise when walking at a rate of 5.6 km/h (3.5 mph) in an ambient temperature of 37.7°C (100°F) is directly proportional to the level of body dehydration (Figure 3). The highest temperature occurred with no water intake; the intermediate temperature with water ad libitum; and the lowest temperature with water equal to sweat loss[20]. With moderate exercise in normal ambient temperature, core temperature increases by 0.1°C for each 1% decrease in body water content[8]. This exercise hyperthermic response can be detected with as little as a 1% loss (500 ml) of body water[6], emphasizing the sensitivity of the interaction. The predominate cause of exercise

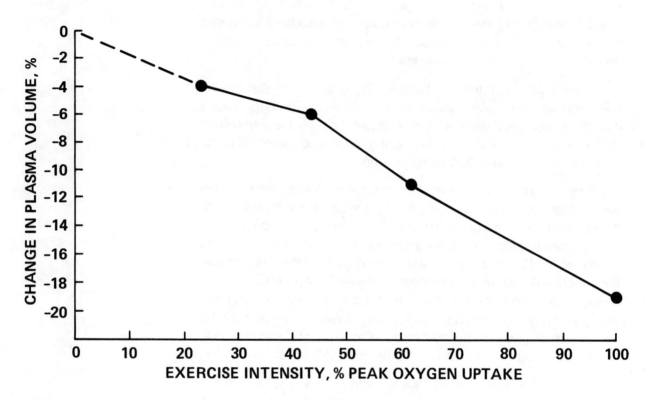

FIGURE 2. Plasma volume loss (shift) with increasing intensity of exercise.

TABLE 4. Change in plasma volume during stress.

Active Stress

Reference	Control Period % Δ	Peak Exercise % Δ	Σ % Δ
Van Beaumont et al.[25]			
3 ∕ Upright, Cycle		-14.9	-14.9
3 ∕ Upright, Cycle		-15.1	-15.1
Van Beaumont et al.[27]			
6 ∕ Upright, Cycle		-15.6	-15.6
Greenleaf et al.[15]			
4 ∕ Upright, Cycle	-3.4%	-16.1	-19.5
4 ∕ Supine, Cycle	+0.8%	-17.6	-16.8

Passive Stress

Reference	Bed Rest % Δ	+G$_z$ Acceleration % Δ	Σ % Δ
Greenleaf et al.[14]			
3.2 g/min			
8 ∕ Bed Rest 1 (ITE)	-6.8	-10.6	-17.4
8 ∕ Bed Rest 2 (ITE)	-6.5	-11.9	-18.4
Van Beaumont et al.[26]			
3.2 g/min			
7 ∕ Bed Rest 1 (NOE)	-12.6	-6.3	-18.9
7 ∕ Bed Rest 2 (IME)	-11.3	-6.3	-17.6
7 ∕ Bed Rest 3 (ITE)	-7.8	-7.1	-14.9
Greenleaf et al.[13]			
3.0 g/min			
12 ⁰ Bed Rest 1 (NOE)	-12.6	-4.1	-16.7

NOE, no exercise; ITE, isotonic exercise; IME, isometric exercise.

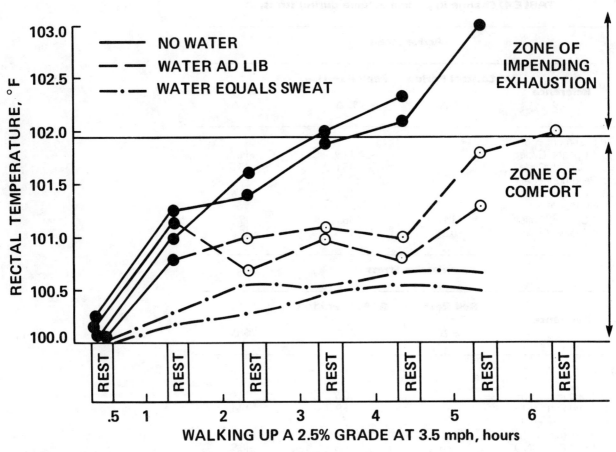

FIGURE 3. Effect of water consumption on rectal temperature while walking in the heat (T_a = 37.7°C, rh = 40%). From[20] with permission.

dehydration hyperthermia is reduction in sweating and evaporative heat loss[8].

Trained athletes, who are able to work at high work loads for prolonged periods, will necessarily have high sweat rates. Unless the environment is extremely dry, much of the sweat formed on the skin of these athletes will not be evaporated; instead it will drip or run off the body, and will not contribute to the dissipation of heat. This situation, and the observation that people working in the heat do not voluntarily drink enough fluid to maintain their body weight, have prompted some coaches and trainers to conclude that fluids can be restricted with no adverse effects. They overlook the fact that the plasma (blood) volume is reduced because of the increased blood pressure, and continues to decrease when fluid intake does not equal fluid outgo. The progressive reduction in blood volume will not only reduce the efficiency of the cardiovascular system to transport oxygen, but will also reduce the ability to transport heat from the working muscles to the skin. Even a sufficient volume of sweat on the skin cannot dissipate heat that does not arrive. The range of plasma volume depletion at the limit of performance appears to be 15%-20% (530-700 ml) (Table 4). The interesting generalization is that it does not seem to matter how the volume is depleted; for example, whether the stress is active (peak exercise) or passive (head-to-foot acceleration). Sitting relatively motionless for 1 h results in a 6%-7% loss (220 ml) of plasma volume[10]. An underfilled circulatory system will reduce its volume by vasoconstriction. In this case, since the working muscles take priority for the remaining blood plasma, heat transport falters, heat dissipation is reduced, and core temperature rises. Heat exhaustion (perhaps with syncope) is the inevitable result. There is no known scientific evidence to suggest that the body can adapt to successive periods of dehydration. Withholding needed fluids will only hasten deterioration of physical and mental performance (Figure 4). In fact, people undergoing intensive exercise training will require progressively greater fluid intake to compensate for the increased sweating that results from the training or acclimation.

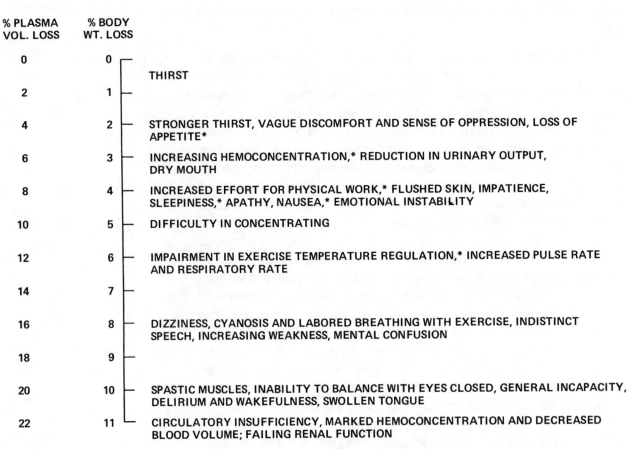

% PLASMA VOL. LOSS	% BODY WT. LOSS	
0	0	
		THIRST
2	1	
4	2	STRONGER THIRST, VAGUE DISCOMFORT AND SENSE OF OPPRESSION, LOSS OF APPETITE*
6	3	INCREASING HEMOCONCENTRATION,* REDUCTION IN URINARY OUTPUT, DRY MOUTH
8	4	INCREASED EFFORT FOR PHYSICAL WORK,* FLUSHED SKIN, IMPATIENCE, SLEEPINESS,* APATHY, NAUSEA,* EMOTIONAL INSTABILITY
10	5	DIFFICULTY IN CONCENTRATING
12	6	IMPAIRMENT IN EXERCISE TEMPERATURE REGULATION,* INCREASED PULSE RATE AND RESPIRATORY RATE
14	7	
16	8	DIZZINESS, CYANOSIS AND LABORED BREATHING WITH EXERCISE, INDISTINCT SPEECH, INCREASING WEAKNESS, MENTAL CONFUSION
18	9	
20	10	SPASTIC MUSCLES, INABILITY TO BALANCE WITH EYES CLOSED, GENERAL INCAPACITY, DELIRIUM AND WAKEFULNESS, SWOLLEN TONGUE
22	11	CIRCULATORY INSUFFICIENCY, MARKED HEMOCONCENTRATION AND DECREASED BLOOD VOLUME; FAILING RENAL FUNCTION

* ALSO OBSERVED IN ASTRONAUTS DURING FLIGHT

FIGURE 4. Adverse effects of dehydration.

Some conditions and procedures that will aid physical performance during negative water balance may be summarized as follows:

1. A high level of physical fitness for endurance activity.

2. Induction of heat acclimation in addition to physical training.

3. The supine position is preferable to the sitting or standing positions when working in the heat.

4. Reduce the work rate to the minimum when exercising in the heat. The greater the level of dehydration the longer the time needed for complete voluntary fluid replacement.

5. For optimal fluid replacement during long-duration exercise allow 20- to 30-min rest periods every 2 to 3 h rather than 10 min each hour.

6. Encourage fluid intake equal to sweat (body weight) loss, and slightly more if possible. Plain water and citrus-fruit-flavored drinks, at 10°C-13°C (50°F-55°F) and a pH of 6.0, are usually preferred. Consider ethnic origin and normal drinking habits when prescribing fluids.

7. Drink small volumes frequently rather than large volumes infrequently.

8. Have fluids easily accessible; many people would rather be thirsty than walk for a drink.

9. During prolonged exercise or heat exposure over a period of days, the sodium chloride intake should be increased to replace losses. If in doubt, omit the salt if an adequate diet is eaten. Do not skip meals as drinking is associated with eating. Avoid high protein diets as they can lead to excessive urine water loss.

10. If the availability of fluids is limited, drink nothing if possible for the first 24 h to allow urine volume to reach the obligatory level.

REFERENCES

1. Bernard, C. *An Introduction to the Study of Experimental Medicine.* Translated by A.C. Greene. New York: Schuman, 1949.

2. Cannon, W.B. **The Wisdom of the Body.** New York: W.W. Norton & Co., 1932.

3. Convertino, V.A., J.E. Greenleaf, and E.M. Bernauer. Role of thermal and exercise factors in the mechanism of hypervolemia. **J. Appl. Physiol.: Respirat. Environ. Exercise Physiol.** 48:657-664, 1980.

4. Darrow, D.C. and H. Yannet. The changes in the distribution of body water accompanying increase and decrease in extracellular electrolyte. **J.Clin. Invest.** 14:266-275, 1935.

5. DuBois, E.F. The many different temperatures of the human body and its parts. **Western J. Surg.** 59:476-490, 1951.

6. Ekblom, B., C.J. Greenleaf, J.E. Greenleaf, and L. Hermansen. Temperature regulation during exercise dehydration in man. **Acta Physiol. Scand.** 79:475-483, 1970.

7. Greenleaf, J.E. Hyperthermia and exercise. In: **Int. Rev. Physiol.** 20: Environ. Physiol. III, D. Robertshaw (Ed.), Baltimore: University Park Press, 1979, pp. 157-208.

8. Greenleaf, J.E. and B.L. Castle. Exercise temperature regulation in man during hypohydration and hyperhydration. **J. Appl. Physiol.** 30:847-853, 1971.

9. Greenleaf, J.E., V.A. Convertino, and G.R. Mangseth. Plasma volume during stress in man: osmolality and red cell volume. **J. Appl. Physiol: Respirat. Environ. Exercise Physiol.** 47:1031-1038, 1979.

10. Greenleaf, J.E., V.A. Convertino, R.W. Stremel, E.M. Bernauer, W.C. Adams, S.R. Vignau, and P.J. Brock. Plasma [Na+], [Ca^{2+}], and volume shifts and thermoregulation during exercise in man. **J. Appl. Physiol.: Respirat. Environ. Exercise Physiol.** 43:1026-1032, 1977.

11. Greenleaf, J.E., K.-E. Olsson, and B. Saltin. Muscle glycogen content and its significance for the water content of the body. **Acta Physiol. Scand.** suppl. 330:86, 1969.

12. Greenleaf, J.E. and F. Sargent, II. Voluntary dehydration in man. **J. Appl. Physiol.** 20:719-724, 1965.

13. Greenleaf, J.E., H.O. Stinnett, G.L. Davis, J. Kollias, and E.M. Bernauer. Fluid and electrolyte shifts in women during +Gz acceleration after 15 days bed rest. **J. Appl. Physiol.: Respirat. Environ. Exercise Physiol.** 42:67-73, 1977.

14. Greenleaf, J.E., W. Van Beaumont, E.M. Bernauer, R.F. Haines, H. Sandler, R.W. Staley, H.L. Young, and J.W. Yusken. Effects of rehydration on +Gz tolerance after 14-days bed rest. **Aerospace Med.** 44:715-722, 1973.

15. Greenleaf, J.E., W. Van Beaumont, P.J. Brock, J.T. Morse, and G.R. Mangseth. Plasma volume and electrolyte shifts with heavy exercise in sitting and supine positions. **Am. J. Physiol.** 236 **(Regulatory Integrative Comp. Physiol.** 5): R206-R214, 1979.

16. Habener, J.F., A.M. Dashe, and D.H. Solomon. Response of normal subjects to prolonged high fluid intake. **J. Appl. Physiol.** 19:134-136, 1964.

17. Kozlowski, S. and B. Saltin. Effect of sweat loss on body fluids. **J. Appl. Physiol.** 19:1119-1124, 1964.

18. Leithead, C.S. and A.R. Lind. **Heat Stress and Heat Disorders.** Philadelphia: F.A. Davis Co., 1964.

19. Oser, B.L. (ed.) **Hawk's Physiological Chemistry.** New York: McGraw-Hill, 1965.

20. Pitts, G.C., R.E. Johnson, and F.C. Consolazio. Work in the heat as affected by intake of water, salt, and glucose. **Am. J. Physiol.** 142:253-259, 1944.

21. Pugh, L.G.C.E., J.L. Corbett, and R.H. Johnson. Rectal temperatures, weight loss and sweat rates in marathon running. **J. Appl. Physiol.** 23:347-352, 1967.

22. Sargent, F., II, and K. Weinman. Physiological variability in young men. In: **Physiological Measurements of Metabolic Functions in Man,** by C.F. Consolazio, R.E. Johnson, and L.J. Pecora. New York: McGraw-Hill, 1963, pp. 453-480.

23. Schloerb, P.R., B.J. Friis-Hansen, I.S. Edelman, A.K. Solomon, and F.D. Moore. The measurement of total body water in the human subject by deuterium oxide dilution: with a consideration of the dynamics of deuterium distribution. **J. Clin. Invest.** 29:1296-1310, 1950.

24. Sciaraffa, D., S.C. Fox, R. Stockmann, and J.E. Greenleaf. Human acclimation and acclimatization to heat: a compendium of research-1968-1978. **Nat. Aero. Space Admin. Tech. Memo.** 81181, 1980.

25. Van Beaumont, W., J.E. Greenleaf, and L. Juhos. Disproportional changes in hematocrit, plasma volume and proteins during exercise and bed rest. **J. Appl. Physiol.** 33:55-61, 1972.

26. Van Beaumont, W., J.E. Greenleaf, H.L. Young, and L. Juhos. Plasma volume and blood constituent shifts during +Gz acceleration after bed rest with exercise conditioning. **Aerospace Med.** 45:425-430, 1974.

27. Van Beaumont, W., J.C. Strand, J.S. Petrofsky, S.G. Hipskind, and J.E. Greenleaf. Changes in total plasma content of electrolytes and proteins with maximal exercise. **J. Appl. Physiol.** 34:102-106, 1973.

28. Wolf, A.F. Thirst. Physiology of the Urge to Drink and Problems of Water Lack. Springfield, Illinois: C.C. Thomas, 1958.

Fluid Intake for Maximizing Athletic Performance

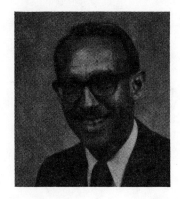

WILLIAM J. FINK, M.S.

Research Associate, Human Performance Laboratory, Ball State University. Leading researcher in fluids, nutrition and athletic performance, numerous scientific publications and presentations. Member of American College of Sports Medicine and New York Academy of Sciences.

It is impossible to speak of fluid intake for maximizing athletic performance without, on the one hand, repeating some of the major relationships between heat stress and dehydration, and, on the other hand, cautioning the athlete against hoping for too much from any kind of drink, whatever its contents. When all is said and done, the coach and athlete must be sure of one thing, **that training and talent are the athlete's best friends,** and no degree of dietary manipulation will substitute for them. The truth of this point is obvious to those fitness buffs who are relatively untrained. When one finishes a three mile jog absolutely exhaused, he knows his fatigue is not the result of needing a drink.

Nevertheless, when exercise is prolonged, especially in the heat, profound changes take place in the body, and two well-trained competitors might well consider whether prudent drinking would give one or the other an edge. Thus, it bears repeating, what has been shown over and over again, that the loss of body fluid in sweat gradually compromises the body's ability to circulate blood and regulate body temperature[1, 2, 19]. As sweating continues, the water portion of the blood decreases, reducing the volume of blood available to the circulation and making it more and more difficult for the heart to satisfy the energy demands of the muscles and the circulation of blood to the skin to transfer body heat to the environment. As a result, the stroke volume of each heart beat decreases, the heart rate increases, the blood flow to the skin begins to fail, and the core temperature of the body climbs steadily toward the danger zone (40.5-41.1°C 105-106°F). In practical terms, performance falls off and the effort of the work is perceived as more labored, even if the subject may not feel particularly hot. In some circumstances, the rise in body temperature can be life threatening.

In view of this, it is important to reflect on how much water can be lost through sweating. It is more than most people imagine and depends not only on the environmental conditions (heat, humidity, wind, a radiant sun, etc.), but on the rate of energy production (work intensity) and the idiosyncracies of the individual[3]. Some people simply sweat more than others. A marathoner may produce sweat losses in excess of 6 liters (2.8 1/hr), amounting to 6-8% of his body weight and a 13-21% loss of water from the blood[3]. More normally, an athlete will lose from 2-4% of his body weight in from the extracellular space. Of the extracellular space, about 40% of water loss comes from the interstitial space (the spaces between tissue cells) and 10% from the plasma volume [4].

It is helpful to visualize these losses in terms of the volume of water one would have to drink to replace them. A 4% loss of body water in a 150 lb. man is a loss of 6 lbs., which is equivalent to 3 qts. of water. It is not uncommon for such a man, if he were running, to lose half a pound a mile from the first hour of running in a hot environment. That would amount to an 8 oz. glass of water every mile, or every 6-8 min. As one becomes more dehydrated, sweating is reduced and thermal regulation becomes more of a problem[4,19].

The effect of dehydration is most noticeable in endurance exercise where the continuous circulation of blood is critical to meet energy demands at a high level. In a recent study (unpublished), we examined the effect on running performance of a 2-3% body weight loss (an average decrease in plasma volume of 10.6%) on randomized time trials at 1500 m, 5000 m, and 10,000 m. In order to avoid the fatigue of previous exercise or heat stress, the dehydration was produced by a diuretic which eliminated water primarily from the extracellular spaces. The results showed a significant decrement in running velocity at all distances in the dehydrated condition and compared to a normally hydrated control, ranging from 3.1% at 1500 m to 6-7% at 5000 m and 10,000 m.

Several studies[5, 6, 21, 22, 23], have shown that efforts at prehydration or overhydration (drinking as large volume of water, up to 2-3 l, either before the start of exercise, or during exercise so that more water is consumed than is actually lost in sweat) have produced favorable physiological responses to exercise as evidenced by a better maintenance of blood volume, stroke volumes, and lower heart rates; and temperature regulation is a least as good as normal hydration when compared to the effects of dehydration.

Without question, therefore, the primary need of the sweating athlete is to replace the water lost in sweat, and, as we have seen, this can be a considerable volume. Chances are, however, that most athletes, for a variety of reasons, will not want to drink this much fluid. The thirst response in humans is blunted considerably during and immediately after vigorous exercise[7], and the conditions of competition often make it impractical to drink as much as one ideally should. A typical example would be that of the winner of a local swim-bike-run endurathon, who, after nearly four hours of work in 80°F heat, and after consuming about half a gallon of water during the event, had still lost 5.6% of his body weight and was down about a gallon of water. Should he, and could he, have drunk more? That is hard to say. Research, however, indicates that the amount he did drink was at least to his advantage, if not critical to his performance.

ELECTROLYTE LOSSES

Water, of course, is not the only component of sweat. Much attention has been given to the loss of electrolytes (ions, salts) in sweating, not only because they are essential for carrying on a variety of important physiological functions (e.g., the excitability of nerve, muscle and cardiac tissue), but also because of the popular notion that the athlete should be replacing what he is losing in sweat while he is losing it, or at least shortly afterward. In practice, however, it is impossible to replace lost electrolytes in this way. The main reason for this is that most individuals will lose enough salt in their sweat to require a rather salty drink for replacement. On the average, whole body sweat will contain 40-60 mmol/l sodium (90.92-1.38g) and 30-50 mmol/l chloride (1.05-1.75g), which is roughly equivalent to 2.3-3.4 grams of salt per liter. As we have seen, the replacement of water alone during exercise usually falls far short of what is lost. T in sweat, and in the case of the more concentrated drinks, athletes prefer to dilute these even more.

Of all the minerals lost in sweat, sodium ($Na+$) and chloride ($Cl-$) are by far the most abundant. In the physiology of body fluids, $Na+$ and $Cl-$ are the ions primarily responsible for maintaining the water content of the extracellular space (i.e., interstitial and plasma water). This is principally accomplished by maintaining a constant relationship between the number of ions and water molecules. If, for example, a great quantity of $Na+$ and $C-$ were lost in sweat, the body could lose part of its control over the distribution and volume of extracellular water. If ions are lost, attempts are made to redistribute water in an effort to maintain the original water-ion relationship. Over a period of time, a severe sodium chloride depletion would lead to a progressive water loss from the extracellular compartment, and therefore from the plasma volume, which may be severe enough to produce circulatory failure. Of course, as we have seen, the same danger exists from acute large losses of water during prolonged exercise.

The long term (3-4 days)[8] results of sodium chloride starvation, however, are not what threaten an athlete during exercise as we normally know it. Under the influence of the hormone aldosterone, the kidneys and the sweat glands are able to conserve Na^+ when it is in short supply, and in fact, one of the effects of daily strenuous exercise is to keep the levels of aldosterone elevated[8]. Although it is possible under the severest conditions to lose up to 12 liters of water and 20-30 g of salt (NaCl) in one day, the normal losses of water and salt during training and competition are usually much less. In one study, subjects were required to lose 3% of their body weight (2.2 kg) each of five successive days by running and cycling and to eat and drink **ad libitum.** The intake and losses of water, sodium, potassium, and chloride were measured throughout the experiment, and in each case the intake exceeded the loss. In this experiment, the **ad libitum** consumption of Na^+ and Cl^-, as measured in all foods, was equivalent to about 13 g of salt (NaCl) per day. The excess intake amounted to about 2.5-3 g of salt per day and resulted in a normal expansion of the plasma volume from the water held with the Na^+[9].

Since it is estimated that the average intake in the Western diet is about 8-10 g NaCl[9] (and sometimes considerably larger, especially in view of the larger caloric intake of athletes), one can conclude that in most cases the normal dietary consumption of Na^+ and Cl^- is more than adequate to cover the requirements of exercise. We ought to remember, however, that the estimated requirement for NaCl of sedentary man is only about 1-2 g/day, and the hormonal influences on the kidneys and sweat glands are such that they show a remarkable capacity to adjust the losses to the intake. This is not to say that there is no special need for an increased salt intake during periods of heavy sweating, but that the specific quantity of loss is also related to the quantity of intake.

The normal diet is also adequate to cover the body's requirement for potassium (K^+). Although the concentrations of Na^+ and Cl^- in sweat increase as sweat rate increases, the concentration of K^+ in sweat remains

FLUID INTAKE AND ATHLETIC PERFORMANCE

constant at about 4-5 mmol/l[9]. With an **ad libitum** consumption of K^+ of 67 mmol/day (2600 mg), the intake exceeded sweat and urine losses by about 17 mmol/day (650 mg)[9].

In another investigation[4], we observed that a 5.8% reduction in body weight and a loss of 4.11 liters of sweat resulted in Na^+, K^+, Cl^-, and Mg^{++} (magnesium) losses of 155, 16, 137, and 13 mmol, respectively. Based on estimates of the subject's body mineral contents, we have calculated that this sweat loss produced deficits in body Na^+ and Cl^- of roughly 5-7%. At the same time, total body K^+ and Mg^{++}, the two ions principally confined to the intracellular space, decreased the estimated body content less than 1.2%. Urine electrolyte losses during these periods are usually small as a result of a diminished urine formation and increased renal Na^+ reabsorption[4]. Thus, it is apparent that during prolonged exercise, the only ionic deficits of major concern are those of the extracellular compartments, i.e., Na^+ and Cl^-.

As a general rule, therefore, the normal American diet supplies the body's requirements for electrolytes, and it is very difficult with **ad libitum** feedings to produce a deficit. Nevertheless, it is prudent of an athlete to be aware of his diet and of his daily weight losses in training and competition. It has also been wisely suggested that athletes of equatorial nations who are accustomed to a diet much lower in salt than the American diet ought to give due attention to these conditions.

Before leaving this topic, however, it is important to note that even though the concentration of Na^+ and Cl^- in sweat would make a rather salty drink, still their concentrations in sweat are considerably less than their concentrations in plasma (140 mmole/l Na^+ and 101 mmol/l Cl^-). Since, during exercise, more water is removed from the body fluids than ions, the remaining electrolytes become more concentrated, not less, so that relative to the cell's environment, there is a slight excess of electrolytes, even though the total quantity of electrolytes has decreased[7]. For the time being, therefore, the greater need is to replace body water than to replace electrolytes. The old adage that all body water loss is also electrolyte loss and must be dealt with by giving both water and electrolytes is true mainly for clinicaltly, it is necessary to give some attention to those things that enhance the gastric emptying of fluids so that an optimum amount can be delivered to the intestine for absorption into the circulation without producing discomfort. It is important to note at the outset, however, that there is sometimes a marked degree of individual differences among subjects in the way they will empty fluids from the stomach. Some individuals will empty almost all of the given volume of drink within a certain time; others will empty very little. This would suggest that drinking during exercise is as much an art as it is a science, and the athlete should always be attentive to his own experience.

Among the factors that affect the rate of gastric emptying are the volume ingested, the temperature of the drink, and the intensity of the exercise[10]. As mentioned above, the larger the volume of drink consumed, the more is emptied within a given time (e.g., 15 min.). This is true up to a volume of about 600 ml (about 20 oz). Since such a large volume can be uncomfortable during exercise, it is normally suggested that more moderate portions of 150 to 250 ml (5 to 8.5 oz) be consumed every 10 to 15 min. Nevertheless, most athletes will find even this schedule strange and inconvenient, or competitively unwise, and will quickly begin to incur a water deficit.

Cold drinks (4-10°C, 40-50°F, refrigerator temperature) empty from the stomach faster than warm drinks. Not only do cold drinks provide a momentary temperature sink for body heat, but they apparently increase the motility of the stomach to cause a more rapid emptying into the intestine[11]. Work intensity, as a general rule, has no effect on the rate of gastric emptying until it exceeds 65-70% of VO_2 max. As the intensity of the exercise becomes more distressful, the rate of emptying slows (and the danger of gastric upset increases), but during prolonged work at a comfortable intensity (65-70% VO^2 max), the rate of emptying remains quite constant[10].

Perhaps the most important factor that affects the rate of gastric emptying, however, is the drink's concentration (its osmolality), and particularly its sugar content. The more sugar in the drink, the slower the rate of emptying. This is essentially true for all sugars. For example, 15 min. after a subject drinks 400 ml of water, 60-70% of the volume will have emptied from the stomach. When an equal volume of a 10% sucrose solution is drunk (the concentration of most commercial soft drinks), less than 5% will have left the stomach[11]. Studies have shown that concentrations of most sugars above 2.5% begin to slow the rate of gastric emptying as compared to water[10]. In fact, it is suggested that the whole drink should remain hypotonic with an osmolality around 200 mOsmol/l.

This situation presents us with a dilemma because, on the one hand, it is usually essential to replace as much water lost in sweat as possible, and, on the other hand, it has long been the intention of these drinks to provide a quickly assimilated carbohydrate (sugars) for the demands of energy metabolism. The practical advice has normally been to choose weak, diluted drinks when fluid replacement is most critical and to use strong, concentrated sugar solutions when dehydration is less of a threat, as in cross country skiing and other winter sports. Some studies have indicated[12,14] that as a general rule the rate of carbohydrate (CHO) delivery into the intestine is pretty much the same for a range of concentrations. Dilute drinks will deliver more sugared fluid; concentrated drinks will deliver the same sugar but little fluid. Other studies[11,18] have indicated that the more concentrated sugar drinks will deliver more sugar.

Recent studes also have indicated that more of certain sugars can be delivered to the intestine faster than others. Since the osmolality of the drink is one of the factors affecting gastric emptying, it was thought, for example, that a solution of maltodextrins, larger polymer molecules, would empty more CHO into the intestine than an isocaloric amount of glucose. Indeed, this seems to be the case at least at a 5% polymer concentration, but not at higher concentrations[13]. Other studies have found that fructose empties from the stomach faster than equal concentrations of glucose or xylose[14].

The larger question in all of this, however, is how well the body metabolizes the CHO delivered to it in drinks. It is perhaps at this point that the research into CHO metabolism touches the research on gastric emptying. It is known, for instance, that taking sugared drinks soon before the start of exercise (1 hr) is probably not a good idea because the elevated blood glucose and insulin levels will produce a hypoglycemia (low blood sugar) at the onset of exercise, which may or may not be perceived, thus placing an added burden on the metabolism of muscle glycogen stores[15]. It is also usually thought that sugar feedings play their principal role in supplementing the liver's capacity to maintain blood glucose[16], but in the absence of hypoglycemia they do not seem to enhance performance[16]. Moreover, although ingested sugars appear in the blood rather quickly, their actual contribution to the total energy used during exercise is relatively small[2, 17, 18]. Such indications as these would suggest that the practical use of sugared drinks during exercise is not as beneficial as is usually thought unless exercise is truly prolonged, often over 2 hrs for trained athletes.

The subject of drinking for maximizing athletic performance has come a long way in the last twenty years from the time when drinking was largely forbidden on athletic fields to the present time when drinking is universally encouraged. Although the word is out, regarding the value of fluid replacement during exercise, it has not always sunk in. The average athlete still does not appreciate the volume of water lost in exercise and the effects of that loss on performance. Yet at the other extreme, we must also recognize the limitations of athletic drinks. Advertisements for them often promise more than they can deliver. Still, there is more research and development to be done in this area. We need drinks that are more palatable during exercise so that they will encourage athletes to consume more water. This needs to be accomplished without increasing concentrations, inhibiting gastric emptying, or causing gastric or intestinal upset. Also they need to provide a usable CHO without increasing the rate of CHO metabolism.

REFERENCES

1. Claremont, A., Costill, D.L., Fink, W.J. et al: Heat tolerance following diuretic induced dehydration. **Med. Sci. Sports** 8:239-243, 1976.

2. Costill, D.L., Benett, A., Branam, G., et al: Glucose ingestion at rest and during prolonged exercise. **J. Appl. Physiol.** 34:764-769, 1973.

3. Costill, D.L., Kammer, W.F., Fisher, A.: Fluid ingestion during distance running. **Arch. Environ. Health.** 21:520-525, 1970.

4. Costill, D.L., Cote, R., Fink, W.: Muscle water and electrolytes following varied levels of dehydration in man. **J. Appl. Physiol.** 40(10):6-11, 1976.

5. Keys, A., Henschel, A., Taylor, H.L., et al.: Absence of rapid deterioration in men doing hard physical work on a restricted intake of vitamins of the B complex. **J. Nutr.** 27:485-496, 1944.

6. Keys, A., Henschel, A.F., Michelsen, O., et al. The performance of normal young men on controlled thiamine intake. **J. Nutr.** 26;399-415, 1943.

7. Costill, D.L., Miller, J.M. Nutrition for endurance sport: Carbohydrate and fluid balance. **Int. J. Sports Medicine.** 1(1):2-14, 1980.

8. Costill, D.L., Branam, G., Fink, W., et al.: Exercise induced sodium conservation: Changes in plasma renin and aldosterone. **Med. Sci. Sports.** 8:209-213, 1977.

9. Costill, D.L., Cote, R., Miller, E., et al.: Water and electrolyte replacement during repeated days of work in the heat. **Aviat. Space Environ. Med.** 45(6):795-800, 1975.

10. Costill, D.L., Saltin, B.: Factors limiting gastric emptying during rest and exercise. **J. Appl. Physiol.** 37:679-683, 1974.

11. Coyle, E.F., Costill, D.L., Fink, W.J., et al.: Gastric emptying rates for selected athletic drinks. **Res. Quart.** 49:119-124, 1978.

12. Fordtran, J.S., Saltin, B.: Gastric emptying and intestinal absorption during prolonged severe exercise. **J. Appl. Physiol.** 23:331-335, 1967.

13. Foster, C., Costill, D.L., Fink, W.J.: Gastric emptying characteristics of glucose and glucose polymer solutions. **Med. Sci. Sports.** 51(2):299-305, 1980.

14. Moran, T.H., McHugh, P.R.: Distinctions among three sugars in their effects on gastric emptying and satiety. **Am. J. Physiol.** 241 (Regulatory Integrative Comp. Physiol. 10): R25-R30, 1981.

15. Costill, D.L., Coyle, E., Dalsky, G., et al.: Effects of elevated plasma FFA and insulin on muscle glycogen usage during exercise. **J. Appl. Phsiol.** 43:695-699, 1977.

16. Ivy, J.L., Costill, D.L., Fink, W.J., et al.: Influence of caffeine and carbohydrate feedings on endurance performance. **Med. Sci. Sports.** 11:6-11, 1979.

17. Ravussin, et al.: Substrate utilization during prolonged exercise preceded by ingestion of 13C-glucose in glycogen depleted and control subjects. **Pflugers Archive, (European Journal of Physiol.** 382, 197-202, 1979.

18. Van Handel, P.J., Fink, W.J., Branam, G., Costill, D.L. Fate of 14C Glyucose ingested during prolonged exercise. **Int. J. Sports Med.** 1(3):127-131, 1980.

19. Greenleaf, J.E., Castle, B.L. Exercise temperature regulation in man during hypohydration and hyperhydration. **J. Appl. Physiol.** 26:847-853, 1971.

20. Saltin, B. Circulatory response to submaximal and maximal exercise after thermal dehydration. **J. Appl. Physiol.** 19:1125-1132, 1964.

21. Nadel, E.R., Fortney, S.M., Wenger, C.B.: Effects of hydration state on circulatory and thermal regulation. **J. Appl. Physiol.: Respirat. Environ. Exercise Physiol.** 49:715-721, 1980.

22. Moroff, Saul V., Bass, D.E.: Effects of overhydration on man's physiological responses to work in the heat. **J. Appl. Physiol.** 20(2):267-270, 1965.

23. Fortney, S.M., Nadel, E.R., Wenger, C.B., Bove, J.R.: Effect of acute alterations of blood volume on circulatory performance in humans. **J. Appl. Physiol.** 50(2):292-298, 1981.

Summary

Dr. John Greenleaf provided a review of the essential role of body fluids in maintaining homeostasis during both rest and exercise. The composition and magnitude of sweat loss during exercise in various environments, and the impact of this loss on temperature regulation and performance capacity, was discussed. The importance of involuntary dehydration during prolonged, vigorous exercise in hot environments was stressed. Suggestions of how to maintain adequate hydration during exercise were presented.

William Fink cited his laboratory's experience studying the effect of fluid and ion losses on endurance performance. Emphasis was placed on the large fluid losses that can occur during exercise in hot environments and the priority for replacing fluids rather than ions (especially sodium chloride and potassium). It was recommended that cool or cold drinks be consumed at a rate of 150 to 250 ml (5 to 8.5 oz) every 10 to 15 minutes.

Fluids which are hypotonic tend to empty from the stomach faster than those which are isotonic or hypertonic. Since increasing sugar content of drinks delays their gastric emptying, when fluid intake is of prime importance, water or drinks with a sugar concentration of 2.5% or less should be consumed. On the other hand, a small amount of salt (sodium chloride) may actually increase the rate of emptying; but salt water by itself is not very palatable.

During the discussion period, the question was raised of dehydration during scuba diving. Some dehydration may be caused by the dry air inhaled during diving, but Dr. Greenleaf also pointed out that water immersion produces a rapid diuresis, causing significant fluid loss. Accompanying this loss is an apparent suppression of thirst, so that fluid intake tends to be reduced. Similar experiences have been reported with astronauts.

The effect of heat acclimatization on the sodium chloride content of sweat was discussed, with emphasis on the reduced sodium chloride concentration in sweat of heat-acclimatized individuals. This acclimatization process is greatly enhanced by vigorous exercise training in hot environments.

The type of activity performed (high intensity vs. continuous) does not have any effect on fluid or ion replacement needs—only the amount of sweat produced and its composition. Since sweat is hypotonic in relation to plasma, it is much more important to replace fluid than ions. In most cases the sodium choride and potassium provided in food, especially at the higher level of calorie intake of athletes, is adequate for replacement of that lost in sweat.

Since the thirst mechanism is blunted during exercise, thirst is not a good indication of dehydration; therefore, should drinks that tend to be "thirst quenchers" be used? Conceptually, you want to enhance the sensation of thirst during exercise, not surpress it, in order to avoid, or at least reduce, involuntary dehydration. That is why it is important to develop and use a very palatable drink that is characterized by rapid gastric emptying. Caffeine increases thirst, and that may be why it is put into many soft drinks.

The issue of attempting to "over hydrate" before a competitive event by consuming a relatively large volume of fluid was discussed. No one present reported any direct experience with this procedure, but it reportedly is used by some European professional bicycle racing teams. However, it is difficult to "over hydrate," because of the effectiveness of the kidneys in regulating body fluid volumes. Also, it is important to remember that fluids taken prior to an event should not contain sugar, because it will stimulate insulin release and accelerate the utilization of carbohydrates during the early phase of exercise.

A question was raised regarding the value of using some standard of weight loss, such as 10% of body weight, during an athletic event to disqualify a competitor for safety reasons. There was general agreement that this was a good idea, but data are lacking on what degree of weight loss should be used (10% was considered too high), and implementation procedures would have to be developed and evaluated.

Several participants emphasized the importance of precautions against increased body temperature resulting from endurance exercise required during the very early stages of pregnancy. A conservative approach to endurance exercise should be taken by women who know or suspect that they have recently become pregnant. Small rises in body temperature, as little as 3-4 degrees Fahrenheit for 10 to 15 minutes, can cause significant fetal damage. Extended vigorous exercise should be avoided during the first four to six weeks of pregnancy.

Very little controlled research has been performed on exercise-induced hyperthermia in pregnant women, or the alterations that occur in thermoregulation during pregnancy.

VITAMINS AND MINERALS

Vitamins and Minerals: What They Are and Why We Need Them

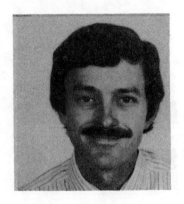

WILLIAM L. LASSWELL, JR., PH.D.

Assistant Professor, Department of Pharmacognosy and Environmental Health Sciences, University of Rhode Island.
Author of articles on the biosynthesis of antitumor antibiotics and the identification of bioactive substances in African plants. Currently studying microbial metabolism of fat soluble vitamins and effects of vitamins on mutagenesis. Member of numerous professional organizations.

The use of vitamin and mineral supplements is frequent in the world of athletics. When athletes use such supplements, they usually do so with the hope of improving athletic performance. This hope is often based on a connection (be it correct or incorrect) between a role that the nutrient plays in the body and some aspect of physical performance. For example, an athlete may know that thiamine plays a role in energy yielding processes in the body. So s/he may use thiamine supplements in hopes that it will improve athletic performance by providing extra energy.

The question concerning the usefulness of vitamin and mineral supplements has been and is still being extensively studied[1], and the results of these studies will be covered in another chapter. In order to decide whether the use of vitamin and mineral supplements is appropriate, we first need to have an adequate understanding of both their beneficial effects as well as their toxic effects. In addition, we must keep in mind the daily doses at which these different effects occur. In this chapter we will examine: 1) the essential functions of vitamins and minerals in the body, 2) the daily doses representing the Recommended Dietary Allowances of these nutrients, and 3) the effects of vitamin and mineral overdoses. Athletes may often consider the use of these nutrient supplements in terms of their possible effects on physiological functions. Here we will cover vitamins and minerals by examining several important systems in the body (the eyes, bones, blood, and energy yielding pathways). At the end of this chapter a small section will be devoted to the essential functions and toxic effects of trace elements. However, before we cover any of these topics, a few points should be brought up about vitamins as a class of nutrients.

VITAMINS

There are a total of thirteen substances now classified as vitamins, and as a group, the vitamins are essential components in a large number of the body's biochemical and physiological systems. Many of these systems play a direct and obvious role in physical performance. So, it is not surprising that the use of vitamin supplements by athletes is a widespread phenomenon. Information concerning vitamins and minerals is found in Tables I, II, and III which list the sources, RDA values and functions for these nutrients. Table IV summarizes the symptoms that are often seen in cases of deficiency or overdose of these nutrients. Two excellent general references for vitamin and mineral nutrition are the texts edited by Goodhart and Shils[2] and Worthington-Roberts[3].

Any work which deals with the use of vitamin supplements should examine vitamin toxicity (hypervitaminosis) as well as vitamin deficiency. Although it still exists, the problem of vitamin deficiency is not as troublesome in the United States as it is in less developed countries. However, serious vitamin toxicities are probably as common, if not more common, in this country than they are in other countries. Many of the cases of vitamin toxicity which are reported every year in the United States are due to situations in which excessive doses are used in the belief that such large amounts might have a beneficial effect for some condition not related to vitamin deficiency disease. For example, vitamin D has been

TABLE I. Dietary Sources for Vitamins and Minerals

Nutrient	Dietary Sources
Vitamin A	Retinol: Liver, Butter, Whole Milk, Cheese, Egg Yolk Carotenes: Carrots, Leafy Green Vegetables, Sweet Potatoes, Pumpkin, Winter Squash, Cantaloupes, Fortified Margarine
Vitamin D	Fortified Dairy Products, Fortified Margarine, Fish Oils, Egg Yolk, Sunlight
Vitamin K	Leafy Green Vegetables, Gut Flora
Vitamin E	Vegetable Oil, Margarine, Shortening, Green Leafy Vegetables, Wheat Germ, Whole Grain Products, Egg Yolk, Butter, Liver
Vitamin C	Broccoli, Sweet and Hot Peppers, Collards, Brussels Sprouts, Strawberries, Orange, Kale, Grapefruit, Papaya, Mango, Tangerine, Spinach, Tomato
Thiamine (B_1)	Pork, Liver, Meat, Whole Grains, Enriched Grain Products, Legumes, Nuts
Riboflavin (B_2)	Liver, Milk, Yogurt, Cottage Cheese, Meat, Enriched Grain Products
Niacin	Liver, Meat, Poulty, Fish, Peanuts, Enriched Grain Products
Pyridoxine (B_6)	Meat, Poulty, Fish, Shellfish, Green Leafy Vegetables, Whole Grains, Legumes
Folic Acid	Liver, Legumes, Green Leafy Vegetables
Cyanocobalamin (B_{12})	Meat, Poultry, Fish, Shellfish, Milk and Milk Products
Biotin	Kidney, Liver, Milk, Egg Yolk, Most Fresh Vegetables
Pantothenic Acid	Liver, Kidney, Meats, Milk, Egg Yolk, Whole Grains, Legumes
Calcium	Milk and Other Diary Products, Dry Beans and Peas, Green Leafy Vegetables
Magnesium	Dairy Products, Meat, Fish, Poultry, Eggs, Nuts, Whole Grains, Vegetables
Phosphorous	Meats, Milk and Milk Products, Carbonated Beverages

TABLE II. Recommended Daily Allowances for Vitamins and Minerals.[1]

Nutrient	For a 155 lb. Man 23-50 Years Old	For a 129 lb. Woman 23-50 Years Old	For a Pregnant Woman
Vitamin A	1000 RE[2]	800 RE	1000 RE
Vitamin D	400 IU[3]	400 IU	800 IU
Vitamin K	70-140 μg[4]		
Vitamin E	10 mg[5]	8 mg	10 mg
Vitamin C	60 mg	60 mg	80 mg
Thiamine (B$_1$)	1.4 mg	1.0 mg	1.4 mg
Riboflavin (B$_2$)	1.6 mg	1.2 mg	1.5 mg
Niacin	18 mg	13 mg	15 mg
Pyridoxine (B$_6$)	2.2 mg	2.0 mg	2.6 mg
Folic Acid	400 μg	400 μg	800 μg
Cyanocobalamin (B$_{12}$)	3 μg	3 μg	4 μg
Biotin		100-200 μg	
Pantothenic Acid		4-7 mg	
Calcium	800 mg	800 mg	1200 mg
Magnesium	350 mg	300 mg	450 mg
Phosphorous	800 mg	800 mg	1200 mg

[1]Values listed for vitamin K, biotin, and pantothenic acid are estimated safe and adequate intakes, not RDA values.
[2]1 RE (1 retinol equivalent) = 1 μg retinol or 6 μg dietary carotene
[3]1 IU (1 International Unit) = 10 μg vitamin D.
[4]μg = microgram
[5]mg = milligram

TABLE III. Functions of Vitamins and Minerals.

Nutrient	Physiological and Biochemical Functions
Vitamin A	Promotion of Growth, Maintenance of Reproduction, Maintenance of Epithelial Tissues
Vitamin D	Stimulation of Calcium Absorption Through the Intestine, Maintenance of Adequate Levels of Calcium in the Body
Vitamin E	Prevents Peroxidation of Fats and Other Substances
Vitamin K	Participates in Blood Clotting
Vitamin C	Participates in Blood Clotting (?) and Collagen Formation
Thiamine	Participates in Energy Metabolism, Essential to Proper Nerve Cell Function (?)
Riboflavin	Participates in Energy Metabolism and a Variety of other Biochemical Reactions
Niacin	Participates in Energy Metabolism and a Variety of other Biochemical Reactions
Pyridoxine	Participates in Reactions Involved in Amino Acid Metabolism Including Production of Neurotransmitters and Heme
Folic Acid	Essential for a Great Many Biochemical Reactions Including One of Those Involved in DNA Synthesis and Therefore Cell Reproduction.
Cyanocobolamin	Essential for the Production of a Variety of Substances Including Some Which Are Components of Nerve Cell Membranes
Biotin	Involved in a Number of Diverse Pathways Including Fatty Acid Production
Pantothenic Acid	Essential Cofactor in Biochemical Reactions Which Include Fatty Acid Production and Cholesterol Synthesis
Calcium	Participates in Bone Formation and Nerve Impulse Conduction
Magensium	Involved in a Variety of Energy Yielding Reactions, Protein Synthesis and Transmission of Nerve Impulses
Phosphorous	Serves as a Constituent of Bone and High Energy Compounds.

TABLE IV. Deficiency and Toxicity Symptoms of Vitamins and Minerals.

Nutrient	Deficiency Symptoms	Toxicity Symptoms
Vitamin A	Retarded Growth, Skin Conditions, Eye Disease (Xeropthalmia, Keratomalacia Night Blindness	Increased Intracranial Pressure, Vomiting, Fatigue, Lethargy, Hair Loss Liver Disease
Vitamin D	Bone Wasting Disease, Tetany	Excessive Thirst, Headache, Muscle Stiffness, Weakness, Kidney Stones Arteriosclerosis
Vitamin E	Anemia, Muscle Cell Damage?	Nausea, Fatigue, Prolonged Blood Clotting Time
Vitamin K	Bruising, Petechiae, Sever Hemorrhage	. . . .
Vitamin C	Bruising, Petechiae, Spongy Gums	Diarrhea, Kidney Stones?, Rebound Scurvy
Thiamine	Peripheral Neuritis, Beriberi, Weakness, Moodiness—Wernicke-Korsakoff Syndrome	. . . .
Riboflavin	Glossitis (Swollen, Magenta, Tongue) Cheilosis (Swollen, Reddened Lips) Scrotal Dermatitis	. . . .
Niacin	Diarrhea, Dermatitis, Dementia	Flushing, Headache
Pyridoxine	Depression, Convulsions, Anemia, Dermatitis (Around the Eyebrows and Nasolobial Folds)	. . . .
Folic Acid	Anemia, Diarrhea and Wasting	. . . .
Cyanocobolamin	Anemia, General Debility, Unresponsiveness, Constipation, Hallucinations	. . . .
Biotin	Fatigue, Depression, Dermatitis	. . . .
Pantothenic Acid	Fatigue, Insomnia, GI Distress	. . . .
Calcium	Bone Wasting Disease, Tetany	Excessive Thirst, Renal Stones, Arteriosclerosis
Magnesium	Anorexia, Nausea, Vomiting	Paralysis, Respiratory Depression
Phosphorous	Weakness, Appetite Loss, Skeletal Aches	Tetany, Convulsions

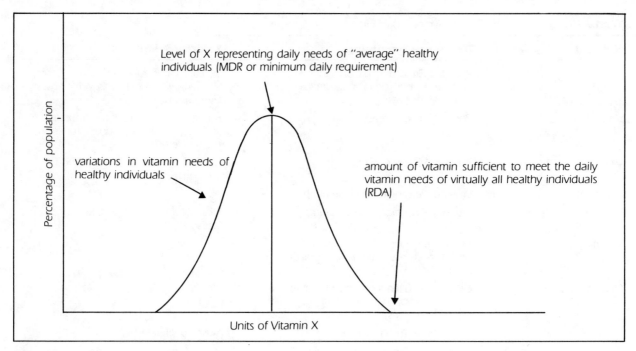

Level of X representing daily needs of "average" healthy individuals (MDR or minimum daily requirement)

variations in vitamin needs of healthy individuals

amount of vitamin sufficient to meet the daily vitamin needs of virtually all healthy individuals (RDA)

Percentage of population

Units of Vitamin X

FIGURE 1. Definition of the RDA.

claimed to be useful in treating arthritis even though that disease has never been shown to have any connection with a deficiency of this vitamin. Although the United States Food and Drug Administration does recognize the usefulness of certain vitamins in conditions not related to vitamin deficiency, these conditions are few, and will be pointed out as we proceed.

The doses at which vitamin toxicity usually occurs (megadoses) are at least ten times the Recommended Dietary Allowance (RDA). The RDA value for a vitamin is that amount which if taken daily will supply practically all healthy individuals with the amount of vitamins needed for optimal health. The RDA value is graphically defined in Figure 1. It is a value

VITAMINS AND MINERALS

TABLE V. Portions of the Four Major Food Groups Which Provide Adequate Daily Supplies of Vitamins

Grains	Four Portions	1 Portion = 1 Bread Slice or 1/2 Cup Cereal
Milk Products	Two-Three Portions	1 Portion = one 8 oz. Glass of Milk
Meats, Fish Poulty, Nuts, Dried Beans	Two Portions	1 Portion = 3 oz. Piece Meat or 1/2 Cup Dried Beans
Fruits/Vegetables	Four Portions	1 Portion = 1 Piece of Fruit or 1/2 Cup Vegetable

which is determined by the National Research Council[4] and is designed to not only cover the daily needs of all healthy individuals but to also provide a significant margin of safety for the majority. This margin of error accounts for the fact that some people never develop deficiency symptoms even though they may have a diet which is somewhat inadequate in one or more nutrients. Table V lists the amounts of each of the four major food groups which are required to provide adequate amounts of vitamins in the daily diet. Since vitamins are not toxic in daily doses equal to or less than the RDA, a person who feels they need a daily vitamin supplement can take supplements in this dose range in order to compensate for any perceived dietary deficiency. However, vitamin supplements are probably not needed in many of the people who take them. Actually the best remedy for a diet which is lacking in one or more vitamins is not a vitamin supplement but a well balanced diet.

Before we begin coverage of individual vitamins, it is important to point out that vitamins are divided into two major groups; the fat soluble and water soluble vitamins. This classification helps explain differences between the two groups in terms of the development of vitamin deficiency and toxicity.

The fat soluble vitamins (A, D, E, and K) seem to have been tailor made for mammals in the sense that they are found almost exclusively in these animals where they perform a variety of vital functions. They have a very low solubility in water and are stored in body tissues (mainly the liver) in large amounts. In fact, the storage level of fat soluble vitamins is sometimes so high that it may take many months or even years for a fat soluble vitamin deficiency to appear in a healthy person. By the same token, excessive intake of fat soluble vitamins (especially A and D) can lead to toxic symptoms. The amounts that accumulate in the body with vitamin megadosing are often much greater than those which can be handled without the risk of toxic effects. Although acute vitamin poisoning has occurred[5], fat soluble vitamin toxicity usually occurs as a result of daily vitamin megadosing over a long period of time.

The other major group of vitamins, the water soluble vitamins, consist of vitamin C and the B complex vitamins (thiamine, riboflavin, niacin, pyridoxine, folic acid, cyanocobolamin, biotin, and pantothenic acid). The B complex vitamins as a group are found in nearly all forms of life and act as essential cofactors of enzymes which are involved in a number of fundamental biochemical pathways. Water soluble vitamins are not stored well in the body. Any dose over the amount which the body finds useful is lost through the urine. Thus the use of megadoses of these vitamins cannot increase vitamin stores. The lack of storage of water soluble vitamins explains why deficiencies in these vitamins can occur in a very short period of time (as little as one or two months). Fortunately, as a group, the water soluble vitamins are nontoxic (exceptions are vitamin C and niacin). This group of vitamins will be of great concern to us since the vitamin supplements most often used by athletes are those containing vitamins such as thiamine, cyanocobolamin, and vitamin C.

VITAMIN A AND VISUAL PIGMENT FORMATION

Vitamin A is best known for its role in formation of the visual pigmets in the rods and cones of the eye. But the story behind the function of vitamin A in the body goes much deeper than simply participation in the visual process. Vitamin A occurs in three essential forms in the body, and each form serves a different function.

There are two major dietary sources of vitamin A, B-carotene and retinol. Carotene is present to some extent in all green vegetables, and it makes up most of the pigment seen in many yellow and orange fruits and vegetables (e.g., carrots). Although carotene itself is not a form of vitamin A, it can be converted to one of the three essential forms of the vitamin, retinol. Retinol is added to skim milk and margarine during the fortification process and is also present in high amounts in various fish liver oils (such as cod liver oil). In fact, the retinol content of these oils is so high that excess intake can result in vitamin A toxicity. Retinol also seems to play an as yet undefined role in reproduction.

Retinol is not only essential in its own right but also in the sense that it serves as a precursor for the other two essential forms of vitamin A, retinal and retinoic acid (See Figure 2). Retinal is the form of vitamin A which

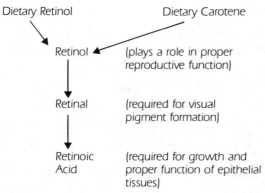

FIGURE 2. Sources and Function of Various Forms of Vitamin A.

participates in the formation of pigments necessary for proper vision. The first symptom that usually appears with vitamin A deficiency is night blindness (nyctalopia) which is due to retinal deficiency. Reports of night blindness have appeared in records as old as the **Eber's Papyrus**, an Egyptian medical treatise dating to about 1500 B.C. Night blindness results when the eyes cannot adapt to low light intensity and it can be traced back to insufficient production of rhodopsin, the pigment present in the rod structures of the eye. The result of retinal deficiency in the cones is glare blindness. Because of insufficient production of iodopsin (the pigment in cones) the afflicted individual has difficulty seeing in bright light.

In addition to causing night blindness, vitamin A deficiency can also lead to permanent blindness. However, permanent blindness resulting from vitamin A deficiency has nothing to do with a retinal deficiency. It is related to the function of the third form of vitamin A, retinoic acid. Retinoic acid is essential to proper growth and also particpates in the maintenance of epithelial tissues (e.g., the skin). A deficiency in retinoic acid results in a variety of symptoms. The effects of this deficiency on the skin are seen when a person develops either hyperkeratosis (skin having "goose flesh" appearance) or xeroderma (a condition in which a scaly "fish skin" appears). Retinoic acid deficiency also affects the conjunctiva, (the epithelial tissue on the surface of the eye). Effects on this tissue begin with a drying and hazing of the surface of the cornea follwed by the formation of small white merangue-like spots (bitot spots). If vitamin A deficiency is allowed to progress far enough, the surface of the eye becomes ulcerated and infected and finally perforates. This can result in permanent blindness. Although vitamin A deficiency is uncommon in this country, it is common in many underdeveloped countries and is one of the leading causes of blindness in these areas. When vitamin A deficiency is seen in this country, it is often due to improper intestinal absorption (which can result from intestinal bypass operations and conditions such as celiac disease[6].

Individuals can suffer not only from adverse reactions due to a deficiency of vitamin A but also from adverse reactions due to vitamin A overdose. Athletes using vitamin A supplements should be aware of this danger. Reactions from vitamin A overdose can come about from one massive dose of vitamin A (see Table IV) but more often result from daily administration of vitamin supplements over a long period of time. People sometimes develop toxicity from taking large supplements of vitamin A in order to treat or prevent conditions for which it has not been found useful (e.g., colds or flu). On the other hand vitamin A overdose can also result from the treatment of certain skin conditions for which it is recognized as often being effective[7]. The irony of this situation is that even though large doses of vitamin A can often effectively treat such skin conditions, they can also produce new skin conditions resulting from overdose (xerosis—dry, rough, scaly skin)[8]. In this sort of situation the individual taking vitamin supplements may mistake these symptoms of overdose for a reappearance of the original skin disease and respond by actually increasing the daily dose of vitamin A[9]. The result can be a serious form of vitamin A toxicity which can cause a hair loss and liver disease (which has been mistaken for alcoholic liver disease). Fortunately the intake of large amounts of carotene (hypercarotenosis) results only in a yellow-orange discoloration of the skin[10] and has no serious consequences. Discoloration of the skin promptly disappears after excessive daily doses of carotene are discontinued.

In closing this section an exciting development in the study of vitamin A should be mentioned. Population studies[11] have linked vitamin A deficiency with an increased rate of cancer. This discovery began a series of investigations which revealed that retinoic acid is capable of preventing the development of experimentally produced cancers in the epithelial tissues of animals[12]. On the basis of these results, scientists have been trying to develop substances related to retinoic acid—substances which have the anticarcinogenic effects of retinoic acid but not its toxic effects. One such agent is now being tested for its ability to prevent bladder cancer in humans.

VITAMIN D, CALCIUM AND PHOSPHOROUS IN BONE FORMATION

Vitamin D

As is the case with other fat soluble vitamins, reasearch into the function of vitamin D has turned up a series of interesting discoveries in recent years. Taken together, these discoveries have provided a much clearer insight into the function of vitamin D in the body.

Vitamin D has been known for many years as the curative factor for rickets and osteomalacia, (bone wasting diseases seen in children and adults, respectively). However, only in the last fifteen years has it been revealed that a metabolite of vitamin D (rather than the vitamin itself) is the agent which actually affects bone formation in the body.

Vitamin D^3 (also known as cholecalciferol)[a] is similar to the B vitamin niacin in the sense that it can not only be taken from the diet but can also be produced in the body itself. None of the other vitamins can be produced in the body. They must come from the diet or from microorganisms which produce them in the intestine. The dietary sources of vitamin D are listed in Table I. One of the dietary sources containing high amounts of vitamin D is cod liver oil, the material from which vitamin A was first isolated. It should be pointed out that most milk sold in markets is enriched with vitamin D (i.e., vitamin D is added during the production process). However, this fortification process is not required by law, and cases of rickets have been reported which were traced back to the use of nonfortified milk.

Vitamin D production in the body can occur when a constituent present in the skin (which is related to and produced from cholesterol) is converted by sunlight and body heat to vitamin D. Vitamin D formed in

[a]Cholecalciferol (vitamin D_3) is the form of vitamin D commonly found in animal species. Vitamin D_2 (or ergocalciferol) is produced from a substance present in certain fungi. Vitamin D_2 is equally as potent as vitamin D_3 and is often used to fortify milk.

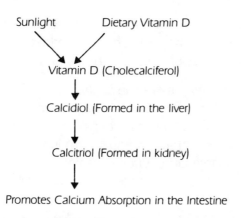

Sunlight   Dietary Vitamin D

Vitamin D (Cholecalciferol)

Calcidiol (Formed in the liver)

Calcitriol (Formed in kidney)

Promotes Calcium Absorption in the Intestine

FIGURE 3. Conversion of Vitamin D (from the diet or sunlight) to Its Active Form (Calcitriol).

this way can and often does account for a significant if not major portion of daily vitamin intake. Children who depend mainly on sunlight for their vitamin D supplies are most susceptible to deficiency if they live in large cities in colder climatic zones, since cloud cover and smog prevent a large portion of the component of sunlight responsible for vitamin D production from reaching the earth's surface.

Once in the body vitamin D travels to the liver and is there converted to a metabolite named calcidiol. This metabolite is in turn transported to the kidney and there converted to the derivative calcitriol, which is the active form of the vitamin in the body. Calcitriol is essential to the body since it is the form of vitamin D which stimulates the absorption of calcium from the intestine. The discovery of this skin-to-liver to-kidney conversion process (See Figure 3) has had an important impact on medicine, since these newly discovered metabolites of vitamin D are being used to effectively treat certain forms of bone wasting disease which were difficult to treat using vitamin D itself.

So far we have been concentrating on the effects of vitamin D on the bone. But we will see now that the most important function of vitamin D has to do not with the bones but with the supply of calcium to the blood.

Bones are primarily made up of two substances: 1) an organic material much like collagen which lends strength to the bones and 2) bone salt which is mainly composed of calcium and phosphate. Thus it is essential that the body have adequate amounts of calcium for bone production and maintenance. But it is also essential for the body to have adequate amounts of calcium in the blood where it is needed to support essential processes such as muscular contraction. Without adequate blood supplies of calcium the body would experience tetany (a very serious condition which sometimes occurs in calcium or vitamin D deficiency). In fact, when forced to make a choice, the body prefers to maintain adequate supplies of calcium in the blood rather than in the bones. When calcium levels in the blood become too low, they are immediately replaced by calcium which is removed from bone salt. The only way that the body can replenish calcium lost from the bones is to bring in more from the intestines by a process in which calcitriol plays an essential role. This explains why, in a deficiency, of calcium or vitamin D, the bones become wasted while blood levels of calcium are maintained, Thus, when vitamin D is given to a person with vitamin D deficiency, calcium supplements are also provided in order to insure an increased availability of calcium for replenishment of bone supplies.

Just as overdoses of vitamin A are toxic, so are overdoses of vitamin D. Vitamin D toxicity has occurred from the use of the vitamin to treat conditions for which it is not recognized as effective (e.g., arthritis). Toxicity can also be a result of accidental overdose during treatment of bone wasting disease[13]. Vitamin D toxicity results in a number of symptoms which are all caused by the accumulation of excess calcium in body tissues. Excess calcium in the blood can exert a strong osmotic pressure on cells in the body. As a result of this osmotic pressure, water passes from the cells into the blood and out through the urine. This continuous loss of body water results in the thirst seen in vitamin D toxicity. Probably the most common symptom seen in vitamin D toxicity (and one of the first symptoms seen) is excessive thirst. Besides thirst, a number of other symptoms can occur with vitamin D overdose. If· excess calcium accumulates in the kidney, kidney stones may form. If calcium collects on blood vessel walls, arteriosclerosis may result. Other symptoms that have been identified are listed in Table IV. Fortunately, the use of vitamin D supplements in athletes is uncommon.

Calcium and Phosphorous

In the previous section it was pointed out that there were a number of essential functions which calcium performs besides participating in bone formation. These include blood coagulation, muscular contraction, proper heart function, and normal neuromuscular function. Blood supplies the body with enough calcium for these functions, and calcium in the bones acts as a reservoir if supplies in the blood run low. In keeping with its function as a calcium storage site, the bone contains 99% of the calcium in the body.

It is important for the body not only to maintain enough calcium in the blood but also to prevent the accumulation of excess calcium in the blood. To this end the body has developed an elaborate system in which calcitriol, as well as two other hormones (calcitonin and the parathyroid hormone), interact to keep the levels of calcium in the blood within a narrow range[2].

Many nutrition experts are concerned about the possibility of inadequate intake of calcium in a large fraction of the population. This concern is based primarily on the high phosphorous intake of many people in this country. The dietary sources of phosphorous are listed in Table I. Phosphorous is another essential mineral which is primarily stored in bone. Although phosphorous plays a crucial role in bone formation, it has other important functions as well. These include modifying the acid-base balance in the blood and acting as a form of energy storage and transfer when bound to carbon compounds in the body. Animal studies have shown that calcium balance can be maintained at a phosphorous:calcium ratio of 2:1. However, negative calcium balance results if phosphorous intake is increased so that this ratio rises above 2:1. Negative calcium balance occurs when calcium losses exceed calcium intake. Thus the net result of this shift in intake ratio is a loss of calcium from bone salt. Whether or not such a loss of bone salt occurs in humans as well is difficult to say, but the phosphorous:calcium intake ratio in human diets is often considerably higher than 2:1.

Other constituents in the diet can also cause calcium depletion when taken in excessive amounts. Chief among these food constituents is protein. There is no question that high protein diets can increase the loss of calcium through the urine[14]. Up to a certain point the loss of calcium can be overcome by increasing calcium intake. But the effects that high protein diets have on increasing calcium loss are difficult to overcome at high levels of protein intake. Certain other factors in the diet (fiber and phytates) can bind calcium and prevent its absorption. Although these substances could potentially cause calcium depletion, the amount required to have significant effects could probably be met only with a very unusual diet.

In addition to dietary constituents, a number of other factors can increase the need for calcium including pregnancy, lactation, and immobilization. Studies have demonstrated that bed-ridden patients have a negative calcium balance[15]. Part of the cause for the loss of calcium in these patients seems to be the absence of the effect of gravity on the limbs.[16]

THE BLOOD, VITAMIN K, VITAMIN B₁₂, FOLIC ACID AND IRON

Vitamin K

Vitamin D is not the only vitamin related in some way to the function of calcium in the body. Recent research has shown that vitamin K is essential for the formation of calcium binding proteins which seem to play a role in bone formation[17]. But an even better known and well established role of vitamin K is in blood coagulation. In fact, the name vitamin K is derived from Koagulation vitamin, the name given to it by the Dutch scientist Dam who first produced vitamin K deficiency in chicks. Vitamin K (found primarily in green leafy vegetables) is required for the production of proteins essential to the process of blood clot formation. For this reason a deficiency of vitamin K leads to very easy bruising and the formation of small red spots all over the surface of the body. These spots, known as petechiae spots, are due to small hemorrhages in capillaries just under the skin. Extreme deficiency in vitamin K may lead to death from excessive hemorrhaging.

People who are most susceptible to vitamin K deficiency are newborn infants and individuals on antibiotic therapy. Certain antibiotics are capable of killing microorganisms in the gut which are responsible for the production of part of the body's daily supplies of the vitamin.

Excessive use of vitamin K has in itself not been known to lead to serious toxicity. However, relatively large intake of vitamin K can antagonize the therapeutic effects of certain anticoagulant drugs[18]. Such drugs are used to treat and prevent cardiovascular disease by preventing blood clot formation within blood vessels. If the action of these drugs is inhibited by excess intake of vitamin K, then the risk of blood clot formation and cardiovascular disease rises.

Vitamin B$_{12}$ and Folic Acid

All of the B vitamins participate in a variety of metabolic pathways which together play a crucial role in the proper functioning of the cell. Many of these paths intersect at various points and in some cases are dependent on one another to operate properly. Therefore, it is not surprising that the level of activity of a vitamin in one pathway can effect the level of function of another vitamin in an intersecting pathway. The effect that a deficiency in vitamin B$_{12}$ has on folic acid is an example of a situation in which a deficiency in one vitamin can cause a deficiency in another simply because the two vitamins participate in the operation of intersecting pathways.

Folic Acid

Folic acid plays an important role in cell division and multiplication, and deficiency in folic acid can slow the process of cell division. In folic acid deficiency the first cells that are affected are those which divide rapidly. Red blood cells (RBCs) are one such class of cells. At a certain stage in their growth cycle RBCs normally divide to produce two daughter cells. Folic acid plays a role in the production of new DNA which is required to make new genetic material for these daughter cells. In a folic acid deficiency some of the RBCs will fail to divide and continue to grow. These cells form larger cells (megaloblasts) which can only survive for a certain period of time. The eventual result is a gradual decrease in the total number of RBCs in the blood. This form of anemia, like other types of anemia, will cause a reduction of oxygen binding capacity in the blood and adversely affect physical performance.

Folic acid deficiency also affects other types of rapidly dividing cells. The cells on the surface of the intestine are constantly dividing and the effects of folic acid on these cells can cause diarrhea which is a very serious sign of vitamin deficiency. Cancerous cells are also quite sensitive to folic acid deficiencies. One popular anticancer agent, methotrexate, kills tumor cells by causing a severe folic acid deficiency.

Vitamin B_{12}

Vitamin B_{12} (cyanocobolamin) deficiency can also cause the type of anemia described above (megaloblastic anemia). However, the anemia seen in this case is not a direct result of B_{12} deficiency but a result of a folic acid deficiency brought about as a result of B_{12} deficiency.

The incidence of deficiency in both vitamin B_{12} and folic acid is significant in this country. Deficiencies in both of these vitamins can easily become a very serious matter if left untreated. Folic acid deficiency is probably most common in pregnant women and people taking certain kinds of epileptic medication[19]. A deficiency in vitamin B_{12} can be caused by many things, but one of the best known causes is a strict vegetarian diet (i.e., a diet which excludes eggs and milk as well as all other animal products). B_{12} is present only in animal foods. Folic acid, on the other hand, is not present in meats but is abundant in vegetables.

The use of large amounts of vitamin B_{12} (as much as 1000 mg at a time) is not unheard of in athletics. Apparently one reason for its use is the assumption that use of large amounts of B_{12} in a healthy person may further improve his/her performance by improving oxygen binding capacity in the blood[1].

Iron

Although iron is the most abundant heavy metal on earth, deficiency in iron is a common occurrence in the world today. In fact iron deficiency is the most common cause of anemia worldwide. The unusual feature about iron deficiency is that it is common in developed countries as well as underdeveloped ones. This fact, as we shall see shortly, is probably due to factors which affect both the loss of iron from the body and the availability of iron in the diet.

Iron is actually present in the body in four forms. The form with which we are all familiar is the one in which iron is bound to the porphyrin pigment heme as part of hemoglobin. An iron deficiency results in insufficient amounts of hemoglobin in the blood. This situation causes a reduction of oxygen binding capacity in the blood which affects the quality and quantity of physical performance. Iron is also present in two other functional forms: 1) other prophyrin complexes which participate in various enzymatic reactions and 2) nonporphyrin iron present as an essential cofactor for certain enzymes. Finally, iron is found as storage forms in the liver, spleen and bone marrow.

The amount of iron stored in the body does, of course, vary quite a lot from person to person. In general, iron stores in women are lower than they are in men, and in some iron stores are essentially nonexistent. Such low iron stores can result in menstrual blood loss which can account for as much as 0.5 mg iron lost every day. Blood loss is also a major cause of iron deficiency in underdeveloped countries, and often the blood lost in these situations is primarily a result of parasitic infection (e.g., hookworm). Besides blood loss two other factors can often cause a significant increase in iron requirements—multiple pregnancies and dietary factors which affect the availability of iron. We will now examine these dietary factors since they are of interest to athletes and others who are concerned about their daily iron intake.

It has already been pointed out that iron is present in different forms in the body. Dietary iron is also present in two different forms, heme iron and nonheme iron. Heme iron is porphyrin bound iron which represents about forty percent of the iron content of meats. It is the more easily absorbed form of iron in food. Nonheme iron, a less easily absorbed form, constitutes the majority of dietary iron and is found in both plant and animal foods. The absorption of nonheme (or elemental) iron is affected by a number of dietary factors. For example, the amount of meats, poultry, and fish in the diet can affect absorption of nonheme iron. Increases in the amounts of these kinds of food in the diet can increase the absorption of nonheme iron. Ascorbic acid (vitamin C) can also enhance iron absorption by forming a complex (or chelate) which is easily absorbed. Other food substances can form iron chelates which are not well absorbed. These include EDTA (a food additive used as a preservative), tannic acid (present in tea), and phytates (components found in bran). In addition to the variables mentioned above, the amount of iron which is stored also helps determine the amount of dietary iron which is absorbed. For many nutrients the body has developed a sort of feedback mechanism which allows the absorption of larger amounts of a nutrient if stores are low and the absorption of only a small fraction of the nutrient if stores are high. Thus as much as 35% of heme iron is absorbed if stores are low and as little as 15% is absorbed if bodily stores are high. The same type of relationship between amount stored and amount absorbed holds for nonheme iron.

After all variables on iron absorption are considered, it is probably safe to say that the average daily amount of dietary iron (6 mg/1000 cal) is enough to meet the needs of many people. However, certain individuals may have iron needs that these dietary levels cannot satisfy. This includes not only women in their reproductive years, but also adolescents of both sexes.

VITAMINS INVOLVED IN ENERGY YIELDING PATHWAYS—THIAMINE, RIBOFLAVIN, AND NIACIN

Very often when athletes take a B vitamin supplement, they take it as a mixture of B complex vitamins. We have already covered two B vitamins (B_{12} and folic acid) whose deficiency results in anemia. The three B vitamins discussed now all play roles in biochemical pathways which harness and produce energy. These vitamins could be compared to spark plugs in an engine. They in themselves do not contain high amounts of energy, but they do play essential roles in metabolic reactions which are responsible for harnessing, storing, and using energy in the body. The connection between these vitamins and energy yielding processes explains why their intake has been estimated to be proportional to daily caloric intake (0.5 mg, 0.6 mg, and 6.6 mg per 1000 cal. for thiamine riboflavin, and niacin, respectively).

Thiamine

A deficiency in thiamine produces one of the best known deficiency diseases, beriberi. This disease has occurred most commonly in the Orient among people subsisting mainly on a polished rice diet (B_1 is present in and was first isolated from rice polishings). Beriberi is characterized by a number of striking symptoms including a muscular weakness which sometimes becomes so severe that the victim cannot stand up. This symptom explains the origin of the term beriberi (beri=weakness in Singhalese). Beriberi can also progress to a more serious state ("wet" beriberi) in which congestive heart failure appears. This type of congestive heart failure will respond to thiamine but not to digitalis therapy.

Although thiamine deficiency is uncommon in this country, a mild form can occur in pregnant women. Thiamine deficiency in those individuals may be caused by loss of thiamine through frequent vomiting and results in mild deficiency symptoms including moodiness and numbness or tingling sensation in the extremities. Thiamine deficiency is even more common in alcoholics. In alcoholics a vitamin B_1 deficiency may result in symptoms such as congestive heart failure ("alcoholic heart disease") but will often present an entirely different deficiency syndrome called Wernicke-Korsakoff syndrome. Symptoms of Wernicke-Korsakoff syndrome include mental abnormalities ranging from simple confusion to coma as well as a partial loss of memory which sometimes becomes permanent[20]. The seriousness of B_1 deficiency in alcoholics has led to the suggestion that alcoholic beverages and bar snacks be fortified with thiamine as well as other B vitamins of which alcoholics commonly become deficient (e.g., folic acid and riboflavin).

Alcohol, when used as a drug of abuse, can bring about deficiencies in. a number of nutrients besides thiamine. Chief among these are riboflavin, folic acid, and magnesium. The sources, functions, and deficiency symptoms for magnesium are listed in Tables I, III and IV.

All of the symptoms that have been described for thiamine deficiency probably cannot be traced back to one single cause since thiamine participates in a number of different biochemical pathways. One of the most important pathways is one which connects a basic metabolic pathway of sugars (glycolysis) to a central energy yielding pathway present in almost all forms of life (the Kreb's cycle). The energy present in sugars (such as glucose) is used by first converting them to a simpler form (through glycolysis) from which energy can be extracted through simple oxidation reactions in the Kreb's cycle. Many believe that preventing the entry of glycolysis products into the Kreb's cycle deprives heart muscle cells of the energy they require to efficiently carry out their work. This results in congestive heart failure. Some researchers also suspect that thiamin plays an important role in nerve cell conduction thus explaining the various nervous system disorders seen. The intake of thiamine supplements both in pure form and as part of a B complex of vitamins is frequent in athletes. Fortunately, thiamine has shown no serious toxic effects in humans.

Niacin

Niacin is another vitamin which is associated with a classic deficiency disease, pellagra. The symptoms associated with pellagra have been collectively called the "three D's," diarrhea, dermatitis, and dementia. The dermatitis observed in pellagra is unusual in the sense that it occurs only on skin that is exposed to sunlight. The exposed skin darkens and then sloughs off leaving scar tissue. (The term pellagra is the Italian translation of the phrase "rough skin.") Dementia which is associated with pellagra has caused some victims to be committed to mental institutions under the false assumption that the individual was suffering from mental illness. Pellagra is quite uncommon in this country today, but was a frequent occurrence in southern states early in this century. During this period there were years in which as many as 200,000 cases of pellagra were reported. Pellagra occurred frequently in this area since many people (especially in rural areas) subsisted on a diet based largely on corn. Although corn contains niacin, this niacin is bound to other constituents present in corn so that is is not available to the body for absorption. In addition, corn has a very low tryptophan content. Excess tryptophan can be converted in the body to niacin in a 60:1 ratio. This tryptophan to niacin conversion explains why tryptophan itself was first mistaken for the antipellagra factor—niacin. Unfortunately, a diet based on corn provides only enough of this amino acid to support protein synthesis and other essential functions and provides no excess for niacin production.

Like thiamine, niacin is essential to a large number of metabolic reactions in the body. Among other things it is involved in reactions which harness the energy produced in the Kreb's cycle. Niacin (also known as nicotinic acid) is often present in vitamin supplements as a derivative of equal potency, niacinamide (also known as nicotinamide). Niacinamide is used in supplements because it does not cause the flushing and headaches that niacin does. Niacin is sometimes used as a therapeutic agent to reduce blood levels of cholesterol[21].

Riboflavin

Riboflavin, like niacin, is involved in harnessing energy derived from the Kreb's cycle as well as other energy yielding pathways. Riboflavin deficiency is rarely seen, but when it is, it usually exists as part of a multiple vitamin deficiency in alcoholics. Large daily doses of vitamin B_2 are not seriously toxic to humans.

VITAMIN E

Vitamin E is a name which actually encompasses several substances known collectively as tocopherols. The most abundant and most active tocopherol is α-tocopherol. The term tocopherol is derived from the Greek word tocos (childbirth) which refers to the reproductive function of vitamin

In the Absence of Vitamin E - Oxygen forms Peroxides

Fats ——Oxidation——→ Peroxide Derivatives
(Can cause damage to cells)

In the Presence of Vitamin E - Oxygen is Consumed
Before it can form Peroxides

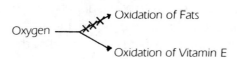
Oxygen ——XXX——→ Oxidation of Fats
↘ Oxidation of Vitamin E

FIGURE 4. Antioxidant Effects of Vitamin E

E in animals. Vitamin E has been called a vitamin in search of a disease, and in humans, this is true. Vitamin E serves an important antioxidant function in the body, but has no other obvious essential role in the human body. Vitamin E deficiency in adults causes only mild symptoms (slight muscle cell damage and decreased viability of red blood cells). Hemolytic anemia often seen in infants (especially premature infants) has been traced back to a vitamin E deficiency.

Vitamin E requirements do increase with an increase in polyunsaturated fats (PUFA's) in the diet. This is because α-tocopherol acts to prevent oxidation of PUFA's by being oxidized iteself (see Figure 4). Fortunately, foods which are high in PUFA's (vegetable oils like corn oil) also contain high amounts of vitamin E.

The use of vitamin E supplements by athletes seems to be related to the idea that α-tocopherol can, through its antioxidant effect, make available larger amounts of fats for reactions which are supposed to provide the body with energy that it can use during athletic performance[1].

Many other ideas about the beneficial effects of a α-tocopherol are linked with the effects of vitamin deficiency in animals. Vitamin E seems to play a more important role in other animals as evidenced by the fact that a deficiency causes sterility in male rats, other reproductive abnormalities in female rats, and nutritional muscular dystrophy in rabbits. These effects have led to speculation (later proven incorrect) that vitamin E could be used to treat muscular dystrophy and sexual impotence in humans. Vitamin E deficiency in cells also brings about changes which approximate some of those seen during the aging process, and this has led to speculation that vitamin E could be used to allay the aging process. One final claim has been made for vitamin E. Some people have stated that vitamin E capsules (containing α-tocopherol dissolved in vegetable oil) are capable of treating burns. Any beneficial effect that such capsules have for mild burns is probably connected with the emollient effects of the oil in which vitamin E is dissolved and not with the vitamin itself. In fact, dermatitis sometimes results from the use of these capsules for burns, and this dermatitis has been traced back to the vitamin E present in these capsules.

Some interesting experimental uses of vitamin E have recently been publicized. The antioxidant α-tocopherol may have benefit in the treatment of certain disorders seen in premature infants. These disorders seem to be a result of the increased sensitivity that these infants have to oxygen. The damage caused by oxygen involves the lungs and lens of the eye[22,23] and may be due to vitamin E deficiency.

VITAMIN C

Vitamin C (or ascorbic acid) will be covered as a separate subject since supplements of this vitamin are used by athletes for a variety of reasons including the hope that ascorbic acid can prevent fatigue, increase performance capacity, reduce muscle soreness, and enhance wound healing. Some surgeons have been known to use vitamin C supplements in attempts to promote post-operative wound healing.

Although the role of vitamin C in the body may not yet be completely defined, it is now clear that is serves a number of functions including a role in the formation of collagen. Collagen is one of the materials which makes up ground substance, a material which helps bind cells together. Some believe that it is a reduced production of ground substance which causes tissues to become spongy in a deficiency state. Bruising and petechiae also occur in vitamin C deficiency but it is not clear why these symptoms appear[2]. Because these last two symptoms are also seen in vitamin K deficiency the two deficiencies may sometimes be confused. One way to distinguish vitamin K deficiency from vitamin C deficiency is to check for the presence of sore, bleeding gums which occur only in vitamin C deficiency. Sore, bleeding gums were commonly cited in cases of scurvy which were reported in European sailors. Although as much as three grams of ascorbic acid can be stored in the body, those stores can be used up at the rate of three percent a day thus explaining the appearance of scurvy during long trans-Atlantic voyages. The dietary cure of scurvy was first identified in the 1500's by Sir Richard Hawkins who recommended that British sailors eat citrus fruits. British sailors eventually came to be known as "limeys" in the 1800's when the use of citrus fruits for preventing scurvy first became mandatory. But this mandatory use of citrus fruit only occurred after thousands had died of scurvy.

Vitamin C deficiency still occurs in this country. However, its incidence is low and is usually a result of a poor diet. A number of factors including smoking and various kinds of stress have been shown to decrease levels of vitamin C in the body. However, these have never actually been reported to cause deficiency in vitamin C. The claims that vigorous physical activity decreases levels of vitamin C in the body may at least partially explain the use of vitamin C in athletes.

The reputation of vitamin C as a "wonder" vitamin useful in treating cancer, treating and preventing colds, and treating certain other conditions accounts for the widespread use of ascorbic acid supplements in the general population. It is important to mention that megadoses of vitamin C can cause a number of problems including diarrhea (called "runner's trots" when it occurs in joggers who use large doses of ascorbic acid). Vitamin C also interferes with glucose testing systems used by diabetics and poses a potential risk of kidney stones and rebound scurvy[24]. Rebound scurvy is a sort of conditioned vitamin deficiency which occurs when a person who has taken megadoses of ascorbic acid for long periods of time abruptly stops taking vitamin supplements. During the time required for the body to readjust to lower intakes of ascorbic acid, a vitamin deficiency results. Rebound scurvy can also occur in infants born to women taking megadoses of ascorbic acid[25].

OTHER B VITAMINS

Vitamin B6

The term vitamin B6 refers to three substances—pyridoxine, pyridoxal, and pyridoxamine. These are all interconvertible and are involved in amino acid metabolic reactions. Since the major dietary source of amino acids is protein, vitamin B6 requirements are proportional to protein intake. This vitamin is involved not only in reactions having to do with the production of amino acids but also in reactions involving the conversion of amino acids to a number of other essential substances in the body. In fact many of the deficiency symptoms seen with vitamin B6 can be traced back to the role that it plays in the formation of such substances. For example, the mental depression sometimes seen with deficiency of this vitamin can probably be traced back to a reduction in seritonin production (B6 participates in the conversion of tryptophan to seritonin). Convulsions, sometimes seen in newborn infants with B6 deficiency, may be caused by insufficient levels of the neurotransmitter **gamma**-aminobutyric acid

(GABA). Likewise, the anemia that occasionally occurs in deficiency disease can be traced back to the essential role that vitamin B6 plays in the formation of heme.

Vitamin B6 deficiency in this country is most often due to the use of various drugs. Probably the most widely used drug which can easily cause a serious deficiency is isoniazid (INH), a drug used in therapy of tuberculosis. INH can directly inactivate the vitamin in the body and can produce not only vitamin B6 deficiency but also pellagra if niacin intake is poor[26]. A secondary deficiency of niacin can result from INH therapy because the conversion of tryptophan to niacin occurs via a reaction which depends on vitamin B6. If this source of niacin is cut off, and if dietary intake is not sufficient, niacin deficiency may result.

Another drug which many believe can cause a mild B6 deficiency is the estrogen component of oral contraceptive drugs. In fact, there is evidence to indicate that much of the depression from which women on the pill suffer can be traced back to a mild form of vitamin deficiency. Another symptom of B6 deficiency which may be seen in women taking birth control pills is a seborrhea-like dermatitis which occurs around the eyebrows and the nasolabial folds. Other drugs which can affect vitamin B6 status are listed with other drug induced vitamin deficiencies in Table VI.

Biotin and Pantothenic Acid

The two vitamins which have not yet been covered are biotin and pantothenic acid. Deficiencies in both of these vitamins are rare, and deficiency symptoms which have been observed are generally not life threatening. In addition, use of biotin and pantothenic acid supplements does not seem to be common in athletes except when they are part of a B complex. No RDA value is used for biotin, pantothenic acid, or vitamin K. These vitamins are provided not only by different foods in the diet but also by certain bacteria in the gut. Since the amount supplied by bacteria varies from person to person, it is difficult to estimate a value of daily intake for

TABLE VI. Some Drug Induced Vitamin Deficiencies

Vitamin Deficiency	Drug(s) Involved	Specific Effect of Drug on Vitamin
A	Mineral Oil	Reduces Vitamin Absorption
D	Anticonvulsants[1]	Increase Turnover of Vitamin
	Mineral Oil	Reduces Vitamin Absorption
K	Epileptic Medication	Reduces Vitamin Absorption
	Antiobiotics	Reduce Vitamin Production By Bacteria in the Gut
Thiamine	Alcohol	Alcohol is Consumed in Place[2] of Nutritious Foods
Vitamin B$_6$	Isoniazid Cycloserine[3] L-DOPA Estrogens	These and other Drugs Inactivate or Increase Turnover of the Vitamin
Folic Acid	Anticonvulsants	These and other Drugs Inactivate or Increase Turnover of the Vitamin
	Estrogens	

[1]Used to treat epilepsy (e.g., Dilantin[R]).
[2]Alcohol can constitute a major source of caloric intake in alcoholics thus replacing nutritious foods which would otherwise be taken with "empty calories."
[3]Used to treat tuberculosis.
[4]Used to treat Parkinson's Disease.
[5]Used in birth control pills.

these vitamins. So, instead of an RDA value, an estimate of daily dietary intake, called the estimated safe and adequate intake, has been established.

OTHER SUBSTANCES CLAIMED TO BE VITAMINS

A number of substances which we have not discussed so far are sometimes claimed to be vitamins (Table VII). However, these are not

TABLE VII. Substances Which Have Been Claimed to be Vitamins

Substances	Claims Concerning Physiological Effects
Choline	Claimed to be a B vitamin[1]. Sometimes used by people in attempts to improve memory[2].
Inositol	May be involved as an essential component in fat metabolism in some animals
Bioflavonoids (Rutin)	Claimed to have Vitamin C like activity.
Carnitine	Plays a role in human fat metabolism but is normally made in large amounts by the body.
Pangamic Acid	A wide variety of claims have been made about the effects of pangamic acid[30].

[1]Choline is considered a vitamin in some animals (e.g., dogs) where it plays an essential role in fat metabolism.
[2]The use of choline in this respect is based on animal experiments indicating that choline may allay memory loss in aging rats[31].

recognized as such since they have not met the criteria used to define vitamins. Vitamins can be defined as organic molecules which play an essential role in the body and (with the exception of niacin and vitamin D) are required in small amounts in the diet. A deficiency of a vitamin results in specific, well defined symptoms which can only be cured by administration of that vitamin. The substances listed in Table VII do not qualify as vitamins since either they are made in the body in large amounts or a dietary deficiency of these do not cause a disease. The case of pangamic acid is an unusual one in that no chemical structure has ever been definitely assigned to this substrate. This point of confusion, however, has not prevented its being marketed. Nor has it prevented a number of claims to be made about its many beneficial effects.

THE TRACE ELEMENTS

Certainly one of the most exciting areas of current nutrition research deals with the study of trace elements in the diet. Trace elements (most of them minerals) are present in the body at parts per million (ppm) concentrations.

Since these substances are present in such small amounts, it has only been in the last two decades that instrumentation has been developed which is sensitive enough to accurately estimate the amounts of many of these substances in the body. A very rapid series of discoveries in recent years has shown that there are now at least nine trace elements which are essential to the body. These elements are listed in Table VIII. As we shall see below, there are a number of very important similarities and differences between trace elements and the other class of micronutrients we just discussed, vitamins.

Many trace elements are similar to the B complex vitamins in the sense that they are essential cofactors in the function of a number of enzymes (called metalloenzymes) in the body. Examples are selenium which is essential to the function of glutathione peroxidase (a component of the body's antioxidant system) and zinc which is essential for DNA dependent RNA polymerase (an enzyme essential to protein synthesis).

Trace elements are also similar to vitamins in the sense that levels of one trace element in the body or in the diet can affect the function or absorption of another trace element. The displacement of body supplies of copper by zinc is an example of the effects that one trace element can exert upon another in the body. Excessive intake of zinc has actually been reported to cause a copper deficiency in humans[27]. An example of the effects of dietary levels of one element on the absorption of another has been documented in cases in which iron medication in infants has decreased copper absorption[28].

Trace elements absorption can also be affected by other dietary constituents. Pyridoxine and ascorbic acid can increase the absorption of zinc and iron, respectively. On the other hand fiber, phytates, and a protein component in milk can all inhibit zinc absorption.

Two closing statements can be made about the availability of trace elements. First, vegetarians may have a unique need for certain trace

TABLE VIII. Requirements, Sources and Functions of Trace Elements

Trace Elements	RDA[1] or Estimated Safe and Adequate Intake	Sources	Function
Chromium	50-100 Micrograms	Yeast, Beer, Liver Cheese, Whole Grains, Meat	Essential to Proper Function of Insulin
Copper	2-3 Milligrams	Liver, Kidney, Mushrooms, Squash, Cucumber, Molasses, Yeast	Essential Cofactor for Enzymes Involved in Hemoglobin Synthesis, Melanin Production, Bone and Elastic Tissue Development, and Proper Function of the Central Nervous System
Fluoride	1.4-4.0 Milligrams	Beef, Butter, Cheese Tea, Chicken, Seafood	Participates in Formation of Bone and Teeth
Iodine	150 Micrograms	Seafood, Iodized Salt	Synthesis of Thyroid Hormones
Iron	10 Milligrams (18 Milligrams)[3]	Enriched or Whole Grains and Cereals, Red Meats, Liver, Dried Beans and Peas	Essential in Enzymes Requiring Iron and and Proteins and Enyzmes Requiring Heme (e.g., Hemoglobin)
Manganese	2.5-5 Milligrams	Wheat Germ, Seeds Nuts, Meat, Leafy Vegetables	Required Cofactor in Enzymes Involved in Amino Acid Metabolism
Molybdenum	150-500 Micrograms	Whole Grains, Meats, Legumes, (e.g., Peas)	Necessary Cofactor for Riboflavin-Dependent Enzymes
Selenium	50-200 Micrograms	Meat, Seafood	Important Factor in Antitoxidant
Zinc	15 Milligrams	Whole Grains, Cheese Meats, Fish, Shellfish and Peas	Essential Cofactor in many Enzymes

[1]Values listed for iron are RDA values.
[2]This is the daily intake estimated by the National Research Council to cover daily needs. These figures apply to all trace elements with exception of iron.
[3]This amount, recommended for women of child bearing age, is intended to cover any needs resulting from pregnancy or menstrual blood loss.

elements since vegetarian diets are lower in these nutrients than diets containing meat. Second, cooking and processing foods can lead to the removal of significant amounts of trace elements from foods.

As a group, trace elements do differ from vitamins in terms of toxicity. Only a few vitamins produce serious toxicity, and these toxic symptoms occur with doses much higher than RDA values. In contrast the majority of trace elements can be quite toxic, and some, like selenium, can produce toxic effects at levels of intake which may be only two or three times that of optimal intake. One related point should also be mentioned. There is a growing body of evidence (most of it obtained from animal studies) that deficiencies in certain trace elements can cause birth defects. The closest link between trace element deficiency and human teratogenesis is an increased rate of birth defects in children born to mothers with zinc deficiency[29].

REFERENCES

1 Williams, M.H., Nutritional Aspects of Human Physical Athletic Performance, Springfield, Charles C. Thomas, 1976, pp. 113-168.

2) Goodhart, R.S. and M.E. Shils, Modern Nutrition in Health and Disease, Philadelphia, Lea & Febiger, 1978, pp. 142-144.

3) Worthington-Roberts, B.S., Contemporary Developments in Nutrition, St. Louis, C.V. Mosby, 1981, pp. 135-333.

4) Food and Nutrition Board, National Research Council: Recommended Dietary Allowances, 9th Ed., Washington, National Academy of Sciences, 1978.

5) Bauernfeind, J.C., H. Newmark, and N. Brin, Vitamins A and E nutrition via intramuscular or oral route, **Am. J. Clin. Nutr.**, 27, 235-53, 1974.

6) Wechsler, H.L., Vitamin A deficiency following small-bowel bypass surgery for obesity, **Arch. Dermatol.**, 115, 73-5, 1979.

7) Gunther, S., Vitamin A acid in Darier's disease, **Acta Derm. Venereal** (Suppl.) 74, 146-51, 1975.

8) Shaywitz, B.A., N.J. Siegel, and H.A. Pearson, Megavitamins for minimal brain dysfunction, a potential dangerous therapy, **J. Am. Med. Assoc.,** 238, 1749-50, 1977.

9) Eaton, M.L., Chronic hypervitaminosis A, **Am. J. Hosp. Pharm.,** 35, 1099-1102, 1978.

10) Josephs, H.W., Hypervitaminosis A and carotenemia, **Am. J. Dis.** Child, 67, 33-43, 1944.

11) Bjelke, E., Dietary vitamin A and human lung cancer, **Int. J. Cancer,** 15, 561-5, 1975.

12) Sporn, M.B., Retinoids and carcinogens, **Nutr. Rev.,** 35, 65-9, 1977.

13) Clinical Nutrition Cases, Vitamin D intoxication treated with glucocorticoids, **Nutr. Revs.,** 37, 323-4, 1979.

14) Margen, S., J.Y. Chu, N.A. Kaufman, et al., The calciuretic effect of dietary protein, **Am. J. Clin. Nutr.,** 27, 584-9, 1974.

15) Emiola, L. and J.P. O-Shea, Effects of physical activity and nutrition on bone density measured by radiographic techniques, **Nutr. Rep. Intern.,** 17, 669-72, 1978.

16) Shore, J.D. and C.F. Consolazio, **U.S. Army Med. Res. Nutr. Lab. Rep.,** 241, 1-13, 1959.

17) Lian, J.B., P.V. Hauschka, and P.M. Gallop, Properties and biosynthesis of a vitamin K-dependent calcium binding protein in bone, **Fed. Proc.,** 37, 2615-20, 1976.

18) Quick, A.J., Leafy vegetables in diet alter prothrombin time in patients taking anticoagulant drugs, **J. Am. Med. Assoc.,** 187, 27, 1964.

19) Wells, D.G., Folic acid and neuropathy in epilepsy, **Lancet,** 1, 146, 1968.

20) Wallis, W.E., E. Willoughby and P. Baker, Coma in the Wernicke-Korsakoff syndrome, **Lancet,** 2, 400-1, 1978.

21) Altschul, R., A. Hoffer, and J.D. Stephen, Influence of nicotinic acid on serum cholesterol in man, **Archs. Biochem. Biophys.,** 54, 558-9, 1955.

22) Horwitt, M.K., Therapeutic uses of vitamin E in medicine, **Nut. Revs.,** 38, 105-13, 1980.

23) Johnson, L., D. Schaffer and T.R. Boggs, Jr., The premature infant, vitamin E and retrolental fibroplasia, **Am. J.Clin. Nutr.,** 27, 1158-73,1974.

24) Free, H. and A. Free, Influence of ascorbic acid on urinary glucose tests, **Clin. Chem.,** 19, 662, 1966.

25) Cochrane, W.A., Overnutrition in prenatal and neonatal life. A problem?, **Can. Med. Assoc. J.,** 93, 893-9, 1965.

26) Griffiths, W.A.D., Isoniazid-induced pellagra, **Proc. Roy. Soc. Med.,** 69,313, 1976.

27) Porter, K.G., D. McMaster, M.E. Elmes, et. al., Anemia and low serum copper during zinc therapy, **Lancet,** 1,, 774-5, 1977.

28) Minnich, V.A., Y. Okcuoglu, and A. Tarcon, Effect of clay on iron absorption, **Am. J. Clin. Nutr.,** 21, 78-86, 1968.

29) Hambidge, K.M., K.H. Weldner, and P.A. Walravens, Zinc, acrodermatitis enteropathica and congenital malformations, **Lancet,** 1, 577-8, 1975.

30) V. Herbert, Pangamic acid, **Am. J. Clin. Nutr.,** 32, 1534-40, 1979.

31) Bartus, R.T., R.L. Dean, J.A. Goas, et al., Age-related changes in passive avoidance retention: modulation with dietary choline, Science, 209, 301-3, 1980.

Vitamin, Iron and Calcium Supplementation: Effect on Human Physical Performance*

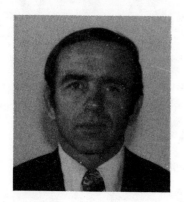

MELVIN H. WILLIAMS, PH.D., F.A.C.S.M.

Eminent Professor, Division of Health, Physical Education, Recreation, and Athletics, Old Dominon University, Norfolk, Virginia.
Author of books and numerous articles and presentations on nutrition and athletic performance. Developed police physical fitness program. Member of American College of Sports Medicine, New York Academy of Sciences and International Society of Biochemics.

*Portions of this paper have been excerpted from:
M.H. Williams. Nutritional Aspects of Human Physical and Athletic Performance. Springfield, Illinois: C.C. Thomas Company, 1976.

INTRODUCTION

Athletes in training for competition are always searching for the ultimate ingredient which may give them the so-called racer's edge. Thus, over the years a number of theoretical ergogenic aids have been utilized in attempts to increase athletic performance capability, including mechanical aids such as heat, psychological aids such as hypnosis, physiological aids such as oxygen, and pharmacological aids such as amphetamines. Since the three major functions of nutrients in food—to build and repair body tissues, to regulate metabolic processes and to supply energy—are very relevant to physical performance, it is no wonder that nutritional ergogenic aids have been part of the athlete's dietary regimen from time immemorial. Perusal of the literature reveals that at one time or another all six nutrients—carbohydrate, fat, protein, vitamins, minerals and water—have been used in attempts to improve physical performance.

Vitamins and minerals are involved in a multitude of physiological reactions which are essential to normal metabolism, growth, and development of the human body. Vitamins are complex organic substances that act principally as regulators of metabolic processes, usually acting as coenzymes. They are essential for the various energy transformations which occur in the body. Minerals are found in all body cells and are essential components of enzymes and other physiological compounds that help regulate such functions as oxygen transport, excitability of muscle and nerve tissue, acid-base balance and water metabolism, to name a few. Since many of these physiological functions are vital during exercise, a pronounced deficiency of key vitamins and/or minerals could prove detrimental to optimal physical performance.

It is axiomatic that a certain amount of selected vitamins and minerals are essential in the diet. Lack of a particular vitamin or mineral could cause a deficiency disease. This was a main cause of many disorders in the past, and deficiency diseases still persist in some parts of the world today. However, in a modern industrial society with a well-balanced diet, outright deficiency diseases are rare. Nevertheless, in a review of studies of vitamin and mineral nuitrition in the United States from 1950-1968, Davis and his associates (1969) concluded that a significant proportion of the population examined had intakes below the RDA, and some of the biochemical indices were in the deficient range. The Ten State (National Nutrition) survey, completed in 1972, also revealed potential deficiency problems with vitamin A, riboflavin and iron, while the Health and Nutrition Examination survey (HANES) from 1971-1974 revealed deficiencies in kilocalories and protein in the general population, iron deficiency in young males and all females, and calcium deficiency in older females (Hamilton and Whitney, 1979). These surveys have been used as rationale to recommend vitamin and mineral supplementation to athletes.

CURRENT PRACTICES

Many coaches and athletes apparently believe that nutrient supplementation is essential for optimal performance. In a recent report, approximately 68 percent of the coaches surveyed recommended vitamin supplementation to their athletes at one time or another (Bentivegna et al, 1979). Approximately 35 percent of coaches in the Big Ten Conference instructed their athletes to take vitamin and/or mineral supplements (Wolf et al, 1979). Seventy-five percent of college athletes surveyed believed that athletes need more vitamins than non-athletes (Grandjean et al, 1981), and the coaches and athletes are translating these beliefs into action. Van Huss (1974) cited a report that 84 percent of Olympic athletes used vitamin supplements. In a report to a United States Senate subcommittee studying the role of drugs in athletics, a team physician for the 1968 United States Olympic team reported the widespread use of various food supplements, including multivitamins, vitamin B_{12} and vitamin E. He also noticed some athletes consuming as much as 10,000 mg vitamin C in one day, and receiving injections of 1000 mg vitamin B_{12} an hour before competition (United States Senate, 1973; Hanley, 1968). Novich (1973) reported that weight lifters consumed prodigious amounts of vitamin B_{12}, iron, vitamin C and other vitamins in the B complex family. Talbot (1974), the assistant coach of the Canadian national swim team, indicated he was not aware of a hard training distance athlete who could be successful without vitamin supplementation or some form of mineral supplements. Nutritionists and physicians associated with various Olympic teams also reported that their athletes received vitamin and mineral supplements (Ryan, 1977). In a very recent survey with college athletes, 27 percent admitted to taking dietary supplements (Grandjean et al, 1981).

Thus, it appears that vitamin and mineral supplementation to athletes is rather prevalent. However, this practice is not generally recommended by nutritionists, exercise physiologists, and physicians involved in human performance. They contend that a balanced diet is the only dietary requirement for optimal performance (Grandjean, 1981).

In an attempt to help resolve this controversial issue, the purpose of this paper is to review the available literature relative to supplementation of several key vitamins and minerals which may have implications for physical performance.

VITAMINS

As noted above, some contend that vitamin supplementation will enhance athletic performance capacity. However, the available objective experimental evidence appears to be rather limited. In the following discussion, each vitamin will be briefly discussed in relation to the theoretical physiological application to athletics and the available experimental evidence relative to supplementation. No vitamin deficiency studies will be reviewed as Keys (1943), in his classical experiments, has noted that the capacity to perform physical work is obviously hindered by the development of vitamin deficiency states.

Vitamin A (Retinol)

Vitamin A is a term used to designate several compounds which are biologically active, including retinol and the carotenoids. Vitamin A is associated with a number of bodily functions, but its major function is to help maintain a normal visual system. Vitamin A is toxic in excess.

The application of vitamin A supplementation to athletics does not appear to be substantiated upon theoretical or practical bases, although Russian research (Anonymous, 1971A) has suggested that in sports requiring considerable eye alertness and stress, extra vitamin A is needed.

In the only study uncovered, Wald and his associates (1942) placed 5 subjects on a vitamin A deficient diet for 6 months, and then placed them on a vitamin supplement program for 6 weeks. Physical performance was tested on a treadmill, with a 15 minute warm-up followed by a run to exhaustion. Measures of heart rate, oxygen uptake, lung ventilation and blood lactate were monitored. In general, during the 6 months of the vitamin A deficiency, no significant decrements were noted in physiological functions during submaximal or maximal exercise. Endurance capacity was not compromised. In addition, no significant effects were elicited during the 6 weeks of supplementation. It would appear that vitamin A supplementation is not necessary in athletes on an adequate diet. Bodily stores are available for short term deficiency periods.

The B Vitamins

The B vitamins are thiamine (B_1), riboflavin (B_2), niacin, pyridoxine (B_6), pantothenic acid, folic acid, cyanocobalamin (B_{12}), and biotin. Although the following are not known as vitamins in the strictest sense of the word, they have been historically grouped with the B vitamins: choline, inositol and para-aminobenzoic acid. The B vitamins are water soluble. The use of vitamin B supplementation in athletics has been advocated by several authorities due to the diverse roles of the B vitamins in energy metabolism.

Vitamin B_1 (Thiamine)

Thiamine, vitamin B_1, plays an important role in energy metabolism and the nervous system. Early and Carlson (1969) indicated that thiamine may modify physiological processes able to deter fatigue. Thiamine plays an important role in the oxidative decarboxylation of pyruvate to acetyl CoA for entrance into the Krebs cycle and subsequent oxidation to ATP. If the thiamine level was deficient, the increased demand for acetyl CoA during physical activity would not be met; hence, more pyruvate would be converted to lactic acid, and possibly fatigue would develop. Early and Carlson also noted thiamine deficiency could result in inadequate amounts of succinate, a co-ingredient of heme. A deficiency in heme would limit the oxygen carrying capacity of the blood. Brozek (1962), analyzing the research reports emanating from the Institute of Nutrition of the U.S.S.R. Academy of Medical Sciences, noted the relationship of thiamine to glucose metabolism, glucose being essential for the optimal functioning of the central nervous system.

The need for thiamine replenishment would appear to be dependent upon the daily loss. As related to exercise, the National Research Council (1974) noted that the need for thiamine is dependent upon energy expenditure and is influenced by carbohydrate intake. They have reported that as energy expenditure is increased during physical activity, the increased needs for thiamine, or any other nutrient, should be met by the larger quantities of foods consumed, provided they are well selected. Nevertheless, Vytchikova (1958) has indicated that the usual content of thiamine (1.5-2.0 mg/day) in food rations of athletes is considered insufficient, and that medical observaters recommend approximately 10-20 mg daily supplementation.

Since the role of thiamine in energy metabolism has been known for over 30 years, it has been one of the most studied vitamins. Even so, the total number of studies in relation to physical performance is limited, and in some cases, experimental methodology was inadequate to validly assess the role of thiamine. Two early studies reported a beneficial effect of B_1 supplementation. With little detail available, Gounelle (1940) reported that the supplementation of diets of bicyclists with vitamin B_1 improved their performance during the Tour de France race in 1939. McCormick (1940) suggested that increased thiamine intake would improve oxygen uptake and sustained physical performance. In an experiment with no controls, no statistical treatment, and tremendous potential for placebo effect, he reported significant gains on an endurance arm holding test after one week of B_1 supplementation.

Several other studies revealed no significant effect of B_1 supplementation on physical performance. Karpovich and Millman (1942) replicated McCormick's study with better controls, using pre-test and post-test scores as well as a control placebo group. The thiamine supplement was 5 mg/day for 1 week. There was no significant effect of the thiamine on the arm endurance test. Keys and his colleagues (1943), in four series of complex experiments each 10-12 weeks long, studied the effect of controlled thiamine intake upon a number of performance parameters, including strength, and responses during brief, exhausting work and prolonged severe work. There were 4 subjects in each series of experiments, and the average thiamine intakes in the 4 series were 0.63, 0.53, 0.33 and 0.23 mg/1000 calories. The results indicated, for the period of time studied, no benefit of any kind upon the physical performance parameters was produced by an intake of more than 0.23 mg/1000 calories. Since the diet was normal except for thiamine control, and consisted of 3000 calories/day, the lowest level of thiamine intake for a 10-12 week period was 0.69 mg/day. For the males used in this study, this value would be approximately half of the RDA.

In a later study by Archdeacon and Murlin (1944), 3 persons were subjected to a moderate exercise workload and a workload to exhaustion on a bicycle ergometer during a period of thiamine deprivation. The subjects were restricted to thiamine intakes of 0.27 mg/day on one diet and 0.15 mg/day on another. The general results reflected a decline in muscular endurance within 10-14 days on the deficient diet, increasing back to normal when the vitamins were restored. However, they also noted that the inclusion of B complex vitamins in a diet already adequate in these vitamins did not result in increased muscular endurance.

Although it appears that thiamine plays an important role in some metabolic processes associated with energy metabolism and central nervous system functioning, there is no conclusive evidence to support the contention that thiamine intake above and beyond normal RDA will enhance physical performance.

Vitamin B_2 (Riboflavin)

Riboflavin, vitamin B_2, functions as a coenzyme for a group of flavoproteins concerned with biological oxidations, the most common one being flavin adenine dinucleotide (FAD). Its role in man appears to be central to the oxidative reactions occurring in the energy schema of the mitochondria, and thus would be deemed important for endurance type sports. Moreover, Haralambie (1976) noted that riboflavin may also be important for the effective functioning of glycolytic enzymes, suggesting that a deficiency could have a negative effect upon certain anaerobic type sports where a high glycolytic rate is important.

Only one study was found that investigated the effect of riboflavin supplementation on physical performance. Potenza (1959) reported an increased resistance to fatigue on a dynamometer. However, there was no statistical analysis of the data. After a rather thorough analysis of the available literature, the National Research Council (1974) and Horwitt (1980) noted that the requirement for riboflavin does not appear to be related to energy utilization or muscular activity.

Niacin

Niacin is also known as nicotinic acid, nicotinamide, or the antipellagra vitamin. The major function of niacin is to serve as a component of two important coenzymes concerned with glycolysis, fat synthesis and tissue respiration. Nicotinamide adenine dinucleotide (NAD) and nicotinamide adenine dinucleotide phosphate (NADP) serve as hydrogen acceptors in the energy schema. According to White, Handler and Smith (1973), no serious impairment of oxidative reactions have been demonstrated in tissues of niacin deficient animals. On the other hand, Bialecki (1962) observed an increase in niacin in the blood of man after a short exhausting exercise. He noted that these results suggest increased demand for niacin in physical exertion. With the role that NAD plays in glycolysis, it might be theorized that increased niacin levels might lead to increased anaerobic capacity.

Frankau (1943) suggested an ergogenic effect of niacin, primarily in an anaerobic exercise task. The performance task was an agility test similar to a shuttle run. Subjects were tested 1.5 to 3 hours after taking 50-200 mg niacin. Highly significant improvements in shuttle run times were noted and Frankau concluded that niacin, given to fit young men, could result in increased efficiency in severe tests involving coordination and physical effort. It should be noted, however, that no statistical analysis was run on the data, and the explicit experimental methodology was not noted. In a later study, Hilsendager and Karpovich (1964) studied the effect of 75mg niacin upon endurance capacity of 86 subjects as measured by performance on either a bicycle ergometer or forearm ergometer. A double blind placebo experimental design was used with a double repeated measures application. The data from this well designed experiment revealed no significant effect of the treatments upon the endurance task.

Carlson and Oro (1962) found that the plasma-free fatty acids (FFA) decreased within 15-30 minutes following administration of niacin. After 60-90 minutes, the plasma FFA rose again. Since plasma FFA are a source of energy during prolonged submaximal work, there may be implications relative to niacin supplementation. In a subsequent study, Carlson and his associates (1963) reported that niacin greatly decreased mobilization of FFA into the blood at both rest and during exercise. The rise in the RQ and the fall in the plasma concentration of glucose following the administration of niacin suggests that increased combustion of carbohydrate occurred in association with the decreased availability of energy from FFA. However, the investigators noted niacin had no effect on the efficiency of work.

Some have contended that the reduction in plasma FFA could contribute to the development of fatigue, since muscle glycogen would be used at a faster rate during prolonged exercise. Bergstrom and his associates (1969) studied the effect of niacin on muscular endurance capacity in two series of experiments. The niacin blocked the release of

FFA, thus the muscle used glycogen for its main source of energy. The ability to perform either short term near-maximal work or prolonged submaximal work was unchanged after administration of niacin. However, the subjects experienced the work after administration of niacin as heavier and more fatiguing. Thus, although glycogen was utilized to a greater degree during exercise, and theoretically has a greater efficiency ratio than the oxidation of fats, the objective evidence did not support a beneficial effect of niacin while the subjective evaluation of the work task suggested a detrimental effect.

Based upon current viewpoints, the use of niacin as an ergogenic food supplement is contraindicated.

Vitamin B_6 (Pyridoxine)

Vitamin B_6 is not a single substance, but rather a collective term for 3 naturally occurring pyridines - pyriodoxine, pyridoxal and pyridoxamine - which are all metabolically and functionally related. Vitamin B_6 is a component of over 60 enzyme systems and plays a central role in the biochemical reactions whereby a cell converts nutrient amino acids into the particular amino acid necessary for the cell's own activities. Buskirk and Haymes (1972) reported that vitamin B_6 is important in the formation of hemoglobin, myoglobin and the cytochromes, all compounds essential to the oxygen transportation and utilization processes in the body. B_6 is also involved in the initial breakdown of glycogen. Thus, one might theorize that B_6 would be helpful in endurance type activities.

Only one study has been uncovered relative to the effect of vitamin B_6. Lawrence and his associates (1975B) investigated the effect of 51 mg pyridoxine HC1 (vitamin B_6) given daily for a 6 month period upon the endurance capacity of trained competitive swimmers. Subjects were matched on age, sex and swimming ability and assigned to the treatment or a placebo group. A control group also was utilized. Swimming endurance was measured by performance times in ten intermittant 100 yard swims. The test was administered 5 times during the conduct of the study. Blood analyses indicated a more saturated B_6 status, but there was no significant effect of the supplementation in comparison to the placebo and control groups.

Vitamin B_{12} (Cyanocobalamin)

Vitamin B_{12} is involved in a variety of metabolic processes, including carbohydrate and fat metabolism. However, the belief in the ergogenic effect of vitamin B_{12} may be based upon its role in the prevention of pernicious anemia, although it is unlikely the normal athlete will have this type of anemia. Nevertheless, Hirata (1973) has noted that vitamin B_{12} injection is a common practice throughout the athletic world, with some athletes receiving 1000 mg about an hour before competition. A recent report (Chase, 1976) reported that John Walker, a former world record holder in the mile, receives B_{12} injections in order to "produce richer blood." These reports are suggestive of an increased ability to deliver oxygen, thus possibly enhancing endurance capacity.

Several studies investigated vitamin B_{12} supplementation and physical performance, and found no beneficial effects. Montoye and his colleagues (1955) studied the effect of B_{12} supplementation upon performance in a half-mile run. Fifty-one boys, age range 12-17 served as subjects. Three groups were formed, the experimental group receiving 50 mg B_{12} daily; a placebo and control group were also included in the experimental design, a double-blind study. The subjects were matched on their ability to run the half-mile. The experiment was conducted over a 7 week period. Although the training groups improved significantly in the half-mile run, no significant differences were noted between the groups.

In another report, Montoye (1955) noted that in normal young men, B_{12} supplementation had no effect on grip strength, heart rate recovery after submaximal exercise, or maximal performance capacity on a bicycle ergometer. More recently, Tin-may-than and others (1978) matched 36 male students upon various physical performance parameters. The experimental group received one mg B_{12} 3 times per week for 6 weeks. Post-test results showed no beneficial effects on either VO_2 max or other standard tests of strength, power and local muscular endurance. Herbert and others (1980) summarized the research noting that the claims made for the nutritional value of B_{12} in situations where a deficiency does not exist are without foundation or fact.

Pantothenic Acid

Pantothenic acid is a factor of the vitamin B complex, and in the body it is found as a component of acetyl COA, the intermediate metabolite of carbohydrate and fat metabolism leading to energy release and other essential reactions. Its richest source, one of the so-called ergogenic foods, is royal jelly, the nutrition for the queen bee.

Nijakowski (1966) reported a statistically significant higher level of pantothenic acid in athletes, in contrast to controls, probably due to the fact that it is bound to acetyl COA and is needed in aerobic activities of athletes. Early and Carlson (1969) reported that a multiple vitamin supplement helped reduce exercise fatigue in a hot climate and theorized that part of the effectiveness could be attributed to pantothenic acid. They suggested that a deficiency in pantothenic acid, which might occur through excess sweating, could possibly decrease the availability of substrate for the Kreb's cycle, thus shifting the energy production to glycolysis, which is less efficient.

Although these reports are suggestive of a beneficial application of pantothenic acid to physical activity, the objective data is not available to support this suggestion.

Folic Acid (Folacin)

Folic acid, or folacin is related to DNA synthesis. A deficiency may lead to anemia. Theoretically, a deficiency in folic acid could handicap an endurance athlete due to anemic effects upon oxygen transport, but no experimental evidence has been uncovered to support this statement. Moreover, the effect of folic acid supplementation on physical performance has not been found in the literature.

Other B Complex Factors

Although several other vitamins and related factors in the B-complex appear essential to man, such as inositol, biotin and para-aminobenzoic acid, there is little experimental evidence to support their use as supplements to the diet of the athlete.

Vitamin B-Complex Supplementation

In many of the older reports, due to the close association of many of the vitamins in the B-complex, the effect of deprivation or supplementation with selected vitamins in the complex were studied together. As the three principal vitamins in the complex - thiamine, riboflavin and niacin - are all associated with the energy schema during exercise, they were the primary vitamins investigated as a group.

A review of the literature substantiates the fact that a deficiency of the B-complex vitamins over a period of time, a few weeks at the most, may lead to decreased endurance capacity (Egana et al, 1942; Keys et al, 1945; Berryman et al, 1947). The athlete on a sound diet is not likely to encounter this deficiency. However, there are those who advocate B-complex supplementation to the diet of the athlete. The research is contradictory relative to the effectiveness of B-complex supplementation. In an early study, Csik and Bencsik (1927) reported an increase in the working capacity of 2 subjects who received vitamin B extract over a 6 month period. The criterion tests consisted of performances on dynamometers and a treadmill. However, a training effect could have confounded the results. Two later studies evidenced no significant effect of vitamin B supplementation on muscular work. Simonson and his colleagues (1942) revealed no beneficial effect of vitamin B surplus upon the capacity for dynamic muscular endurance, maximal strength and other tests involving function of the central nervous system. Foltz and others (1942) utilized a double work period to exhaustion as a criterion measure for endurance to study the ergogenic effects of a number of the B-complex vitamins. In no cases was the total work output greater following administration of the vitamins than it was in the control or placebo series.

In a more recent report, Early and Carlson (1969) concluded that B complex supplementation reduced fatigue which could be induced by loss of vitamins through exercise-induced sweating in a hot environment. They matched 18 high school boys, and assigned them to an experimental and placebo group. The criterion test was a series of 10 dashes, with a 30 second rest period in between; this test was administered on days 1, 9 and 15 of the experiment. During days 1-9, no vitamin supplement was given, and all boys underwent heavy training to induce sweat losses. During days 9-15, the experimental group received a supplement including 100 mg thiamine, 8 mg riboflavin, 5 mg pyridoxine, 25 mg cobalamin, 100 mg niacin, and 30 mg pantothenic acid. Using a sophisticated ANOVA technique with trend analysis, they concluded that the degree of fatigue of the experimental subjects was less than that of the placebo group on the days of vitamin supplementation. They theorized that thiamine and pantothenic acid were the active substances.

Vitamin C (Ascorbic Acid)

Vitamin C is a water soluble vitamin. The National Research Council (1974) noted that the total role of vitamin C has not been completely elucidated. However, it is known to function in the synthesis of collagen, in the metabolic reactions of amino acids and in the synthesis of epinephrine and the anti-inflammatory corticoids of the adrenal gland. It is a powerful antioxidant and also facilitiates the absorption of iron from the intestinal tract. Thus, vitamin C is essential to a variety of biological processes in the body.

Authorities in the area of exercise physiology or sports medicine have advocated dietary supplementation of vitamin C due to certain of its physiological properties. Curetion (1969B) recommended that vitamin C supplementation be increased in athletes during training as research indicated it was effective in lowering the oxygen debt. Horstman (1972) noted that vitamin C, added to **in vitro** solutions of blood, shifted the oxygen dissociation curve to the right. If this would occur **in vivo,** it could facilitate oxygen release at the cell level, thus increasing the amount of oxygen available to the cell. Lamb (1974) has indicated that stress such as exercise may reduce vitamin C content in the body. Thus, there appears to be some theoretical basis for the utilization of vitamin C supplementation in athletes undergoing training or competition.

Regarding the effects of vitamin C supplementation, the results are rather contradictory. Older reports, as well as more contemporary research, are both in disagreement as to the ergogenic merits of vitamin C. Basu and Ray (1940) noted that 600 mg vitamin C daily for 3 days elicited an increase in resistance to fatigue on a finger ergograph. However, when the subjects were removed from the vitamin supplement, the fatigue curve did not return to normal, indicative possibly of a training effect which may have confounded their study. Hoitink (1946A; 1946B) reported that the oral administration of vitamin C for a certain period of time would increase working capacity on a bicycle ergometer, and thus recommended an increase above the saturation level be maintained continuously in order to increase physical working capacity. However, these early studies lacked the proper experimental design.

In more comtemporary research, some reports favorable to vitamin C are also available. Hoogerwerf and Hoitink (1963) suggested that the effect of vitamin C supplementation resembles the effect of athletic training. In a rather well-controlled study, they evaluated the effect of vitamin C upon mechanical efficiency. They pretested 30 subjects and assigned 15 each to an experimental and control group. The experimental group received 1 g vitamin C/day for 5 days. The C vitaminization caused a pronounced rise in the vitamin C content of the blood, and elicited a significantly greater rise in efficiency in the experimental group as compared to the placebo group. Spioch and his associates (1966) conducted a similar study on mechanical efficiency. They measured cardiovascular and metabolic responses to a 5 minute step test. They used a repeated measure design where 30 subjects undertook a control test, and then took the experimental test the following week. Thirty minutes prior to the experimental trial the subjects received 50 mg vitamin C injected intravenously. The results revealed a significant reduction in oxygen consumption, pulmonary ventilation, oxygen debt, total energy cost, and heart rate. The mechanical efficiency increased by 25 percent from 22.4 to 28.1 percent. The authors reiterated the statement by Hoogerwerf and Hoitink that vitamin C mimics the training effect. However, a training effect could have occurred in this study, since the order of administration of treatments was not counterbalanced. Any systematic error in the data collection could have biased the results.

Namyslowski (1960), in contrasting reports from various parts of the world, noted that the German, Russian and Central European studies have indicated a beneficial effect of vitamin C on physical fitness levels, whereas the studies from western Anglo-Saxon countries do not find such increases. He believes the contrasting findings may reflect the baseline values of vitamin C in the different athletes, noting that central European athletes may have had low vitamin C levels to being with, and possibly a deficiency was being removed.

Although the preceding material favored vitamin C as an ergogenic aid, other studies find no beneficial effect. Jetzler and Haffter (1939) reported very little effect of 300 mg vitamin C daily upon the endurance performance of 5 subjects in a 50 kilometer ski race. Using the shotput, 100 yard dash, and one mile run as performance tests, Jokl and Suzman (1940) found no effect after a 7 month period of supplementation of 40 mg vitamin C/day. Fox and his colleagues (1940) replicated this study and elicited the same results. However, the same criticism which was leveled at the early research producing beneficial results could also be applied with the above research showing no effect, as adequate controls were not maintained.

In 3 series of experimental studies of 44 young men under rigidly controlled conditions of diets, physical work and environment, Henschel and his coworkers (1944) studied the effects of 20-40 mg and 520-540 mg vitamin C/daily upon cardiovascular dynamics and performance on standard physical work tasks, as well as other psychomotor tasks, during a hot environment. In general, there were no significant changes in cardiovascular responses during exercise, or rectal temperature, attributed to the vitamin C supplementation. The tests of strength and psychomotor performance also were not affected.

In a field study, Rasch and his associates (1962) conducted an experiment with a college cross country team. The whole team trained for three weeks while receiving a placebo. They were then tested on a distance run and assigned to matched groups based on their times. The experimental group received 500 mg vitamin C/day, while the control group continued to receive the placebo. No control of diet was otherwise undertaken. A post-test at the end of the season revealed no significant effect of the vitamin C supplementation. The authors concluded that the normal American diet contains sufficient vitamin C.

In a study of the acute effects of vitamin C, Margaria and others (1964) administered 250 mg to the subjects approximately 90 minutes prior to a treadmill run to exhaustion. The results showed no significant effect on time to exhaustion or maximal oxygen uptake. Van Huss (1966) also studied the acute effects of vitamin C upon several performance tests including various physiological changes during moderate work and maximal oxygen uptake and endurance time to exhaustion on a treadmill. The subjects were 10 well trained males involved in this repeated measures study. The results indicated, for a single performance, no enhancement of physical performance; however, the vitamin C did aid in recovery as subjects returned to normal physiological values faster, i.e. heart rate, blood pressure and oxygen consumption. One possible shortcoming was that during the phase of the experiment involving determination of maximal oxygen uptake and maximal endurance time, not all subjects took all experimental beverages.

Gey and his associates (1970), in a double-blind placebo experiment, evaluated the effect of 12 weeks of vitamin C supplementation upon aerobic endurance capacity in 286 male officers. The subjects were assigned to either a placebo or experimental group, the latter receiving 500 mg ascorbic acid/day. There was no attempt to control diet, but all officers lived in the same general environment. No significant differences were noted between the experimental and control group.

Howald and Segesser (1975) used two different criteria to evaluate the effect of vitamin C supplementation: time to exhaustion on a bicycle ergometer and the physical working capacity at a heart rate of 170 (PWC_{170}). Thirteen athletes in training were tested after taking a placebo for 14 days and again after receiving 1 gram vitamin C per day for 14 days. They found that the vitamin C significantly improved performance in the PWC_{170} test; however, the lower heart rate values may have been due to a training effect as the administration of the placebo and vitamin C were not counterbalanced. Moreover, they also reported a slight, but not significant, decrease in time to exhaustion after the two weeks of vitamin C.

Horak and others (1977) investigated the relationship between blood levels of vitamin C and mechanical efficiency under maximum work conditions. Two groups of top performance athletes served as subjects. One group received 200 mg vitamin C daily, while the other group used a diet rich in fruits to maintain a satisfactory vitamin C level. They reported no statistically significant correlation between ascorbic acid levels at rest and laboratory indices of efficiency during exercise. Two other studies also revealed that vitamin C supplementation did not increase mechanical efficiency during exercise (Bailey and others, 1970; Kirchoff, 1969).

Keren (1980) recently used a double-blind study to investigate the interaction of physical training and vitamin C supplementation upon aerobic and anaerobic performance. Aerobic capacity was predicted from the Astrand protocol, whereas the anaerobic task was maximal performance on a bicycle ergometer for 30 seconds. Thirty-three subjects were assigned to an experimental (1 g vitamin C/day) or placebo group and undertook a training program for 21 days. Although the training program increased aerobic capacity, the authors concluded that vitamin C supplementation exerted no beneficial effect on either aerobic or anaerobic performance.

Even though the above studies reveal no significant effect of vitamin C supplements on physical performance, one should not accept this as conclusive evidence. In some of the studies, only the acute effect of vitamin C was studied, with little attention to building up the vitamin C body pool. Other studies may have been limited in duration. On the other hand, the studies by Rasch and others (1962), Gey and others (1970), Howald and Segesser (1975), and Keren (1980) with substantial supplementation over an adequate period of time, provide some good evidence against the blanket recommendation of vitamin C for athletes in training.

Vitamin D

Vitamin D represents any one of several related sterols which promote calcification in the bones. The main role of vitamin D is to regulate calcium and phosphate metabolism.

Application of vitamin D supplementation to athletes appears to have no theoretical basis. The limited research which has been conducted substantiates this statement. In a German report, Siedl and Hettinger (1957) studied six subjects over a two year period. Although their results indicated an improvement of physical performance through the systematic utilization of ultraviolet rays, the oral administration of vitamin D_3 did not improve performance on the bicycle ergometer. Berven (1963) studied the effect of vitamin D daily supplementation upon the physical working capacity of 60 school children, ages 10-11. Over a period of two years Berven administered 1500 IU of vitamin D at different time periods to some of the subjects and placebo pills to the others. During another phase of the experiment, he gave a single massive dose of 400,000 IU to some of the subjects. The criterion test of physical performance was the PWC-170 test, a submaximal performance test. His results indicated no significant beneficial effects of either the daily supplementation or the single massive dosage of vitamin D.

Vitamin E

Vitamin E is a fat soluble vitamin, the activity of which is derived from a number of tocopherols, primarily alpha-tocopherol. The physiological rationale underlying the theoretical ergogenic effect of vitamin E is apparently related to oxygen utilization and energy supply, although other rationale have also been reported. Bourne (1968) quoted other research suggesting that vitamin E facilitates the utilization of oxygen by athletes and reduces the accumulation of lactic acid in the blood. Percival (1951) noted that the alpha-tocopherol is purported to reduce oxygen requirements of the tissues and improve collateral circulation. Since vitamin E is an antioxidant and prevents unwanted oxidation of fatty acids, supplementation has been theorized to increase this preventative role, thereby possibly increasing the oxygen supply for other purposes, such as energy production in the citric acid cycle, and at the same time increasing the fatty acid supply for energy. Hence, vitamin E theoretically should be effective in endurance activity.

There are several reports available which support the viewpoint that vitamin E is an effective ergogenic aid, but they are limited. Cureton often used vitamin E as a placebo in his research with wheat germ oil. In one report, Cureton (1955) indicated a significant effect on vitamin E supplementation, in contrast to a control group, on increasing treadmill running time to exhaustion in a group of wrestlers. However, the vitamin E in this study was used as a placebo, whereas the control group received nothing. Therefore, a placebo effect could have been created. Clausen (1971) studied the effect of three treatments upon cardiorespiratory endurance; the treatments were aerobics training and vitamin E, aerobic training and placebo, and vitamin E with no training. Clausen concluded that aerobic exercise and vitamin E appear to be effective when combined, but not when used separately. There are several apparent problems with the study; the level of significance used is unconventional, and apparently the improper statistical techniques were utilized to analyze the data. Nagawa and others (1968) reported that 300 mg vitamin E supplement increased both maximal oxygen uptake and pulmonary ventilation in distance runners. In this complex report, apparently a bicycle ergometer ride to exhaustion was used to evaluate these physiological parameters. However, no results or statistical analyses were presented to substantiate the authors' conclusion.

Kobayashi (1974) administered 1200 IU daily of vitamin E or a placebo to 12 subjects in a double-blind cross-over design. Testing subjects at an altitude of 5000 and 15,000 feet, he reported that vitamin E supplementation increased VO_2 max, decreased submaximal exercise oxygen uptake and reduced oxygen debt. These are rather significant findings and merit further research.

On the other hand, there are several reports, including some very recent findings from well-controlled studies, that supplemental vitamin E exerts no effect on physical performance capacity. One of the most cited reports relative to the ineffectiveness of vitamin E is a masters thesis by Thomas, the results being rather fully reported by Mayer and Bullen (1959). Thomas used 30 young males in a crossover experimental design, each subject receiving a placebo or 450 IU alpha-tocopherol acetate daily for 5 weeks, and then reversed the procedure for the next 5 weeks. He reported no significant effect of the vitamin E supplementaion upon sit-ups, vertical jump, or cardiorespiratory responses immediately after activity. However, no evidence of an overall cardiovascular endurance performance test was indicated as one of the criterion tests, the type of activity where vitamin E may be theorized to be beneficial. Sharman (1971) utilized two groups of swimmers to study vitamin E. The athletes were maintained on a normal diet with the experimental group receiving 400 mg alpha-tocopherol acetate daily while the control group received a placebo. The subjects were matched on pretest performances, and undertook a 6 week training period including swimming and other activities. Criterion tests at the conclusion of the experiment included vital capacity, body fat, resting EKG, heart rate response to a standardized step test, a one mile run, a 400 meter swim, pull-ups, push-ups, 2 minute sit-up test, and isotonic endurance with bench presses. Although some beneficial effects on performance were due to training, the statistical analysis revealed no significant effect of vitamin E on any parameters. Shephard and his colleagues (1974A, 1974B) undertook a double blind investigation regarding the effect of vitamin E supplementation upon the performance of twenty varsity college swimmers. The athletes were matched on the basis of aerobic power and assigned to either the experimental or placebo group. Criterion tests included maximal oxygen uptake, muscular strength, heart rate recovery and EKG analyses. The administration of the vitamin E, 1200 IU daily, was started in the experimental group at the initiation of the intense training season and ended 85 days later. It was a heavy dose, the amount recommended by those who advocate vitamin E as an ergogenic aid. The results indicated no significant effect of vitamin E.

Lawrence and his associates (1975A, 1075B) studied the effect of 900 IU alpha-tocopherol administered daily over a six month period upon the endurance capacity of trained competitive swimmers. The swimming endurance test consisted of ten intermittant 100 yard swims for time. In comparison to both a placebo and control group, there was no significant effect of the vitamin supplement upon swimming endurance capacity as measured by the test, even though the mean serum level of vitamin E increased 162 percent. In addition, the authors concluded the vitamin E had no effect upon oxygen debt capacity, as there was no significant difference between the post-exercise serum lactic acid levels of any group following a strenuous 15 minute swimming test. Watt and others (1974) evaluated the effect of vitamin E upon oxygen consumption. In a double blind study, 20 active hockey players were matched according to their maximal oxygen uptake, and the experimental group received 1200 IU vitamin E daily for 50 days while the control group received a placebo. All players were involved in the same training regimen. At the end of the training period both groups significantly increased their maximal oxygen uptake, but there was no significant difference between the 2 groups. The authors concluded vitamin E had no beneficial effect upon the maximal oxygen uptake of active individuals.

Sharman and others (1976) used a double-blind placebo design with highly trained swimmers matched on performance and placed in either an experimental or placebo group. The experimental group received a heavy dose of vitamin E. Following 6 weeks of intensive training, no significant difference was noted between the groups on a 400 meter swim, an aerobic activity. In addition, no differences were reported on a series of other physical tasks.

In summary, it would appear that vitamin E supplementation will not improve physical performance capacity. However, more experimentation may be desirable relative to physical performance at high altitudes.

MINERALS

Mineral elements may be classified into two groups based upon body needs. The major minerals are those needed in the diet in levels greater than 100 mg/day; this group includes calcium (Ca), phosphorus (P), magnesium (Mg), sodium (Na), potassium (K) and chloride (Cl). The minor mineral elements, the trace elements, are those where only a few mg/day are needed. Biological functions in animals have only been demonstrated for 17 trace elements. The National Research Council (1974) noted that while all these may eventually prove to be essential to man, at the present time only 10 are. They include fluorine (F), chromium (Cr), manganese (Mn), cobalt (Co), copper (Cu), iron (Fe), zinc (Zn), selenium (Se), molybdenum (Mb), and iodine (I). Of both the major and minor elements, RDA have been determined for only six: calcium, phosphorus, iodine, iron, magnesium, and zinc.

The major electrolytes—sodium, potassium and chloride—are discussed elsewhere in this symposium; this discussion will center primarily on iron supplementation to athletes, with some brief remarks on calcium, zinc and other trace minerals.

Iron

Iron is a constituent of the oxygen transportation compounds hemoglobin, myoglobin and the cytochromes. Approximately 70 percent of body iron stores are labelled as essential, and 85 percent of this essential component is found in hemoglobin. The other 30 percent is non-essential storage iron found in the liver, spleen and bone marrow. The RDA is 18 mg/day for females and young males, and 10 mg/day for adult males.

Iron deficiency anemia can cause significant decreases in physical performance, particularly of an aerobic nature, and it is a medical and public health problem of prime importance (Beutler, 1980). Iron deficiency without anemia is also a major health concern (Beutler, 1980; Peterson, 1979), but whether or not it impairs physical performance in humans is uncertain (Beutler, 1980; Pate, 1979). Nevertheless, since iron deficiency can predispose an individual to iron deficiency anemia, the issue is of concern to many coaches and athletes.

In particular, females are more likely to become iron deficient. Due to a lower caloric intake compared to males, they may have a dietary insufficiency of iron, since there is about 6 mg of iron in 1000 calories of the average diet. Moreover, loss of iron via menstrual blood flow, particularly if heavy, may contribute to a negative iron balance. Young adult males also have been found to be iron deficient, presumably due to decreased iron content in modern western diets (Hoglund et al, 1970).

Athletes, especially those in endurance activities which stress aerobic capacity, would appear to have their ability compromised if anemic. Several studies have been conducted with athletes to determine the levels of iron deficiency anemia, and the results do reflect some cases of iron deficiency and/or anemia. Stewart and his associates (1972) noted suboptimal levels of hemoglobin in some endurance athletes during the 1968 Olympics, but they did not attribute this to dietary deficiency. A hematological study of Dutch athletes by deWijn and his colleagues (1971a; 1971b) revealed an occurrence of iron deficiency anemia in 2 percent of the male and 2.5 percent of the female athletes. In addition, another 3 percent of the athletes had mild anemia without signs of iron deficiency, while some athletes had iron deficiency without anemia. In total, they noted that 3.5 percent of the male athletes and 7.5 percent of the female athletes were iron depleted. They did implicate the diet as the cause of the low iron levels; however, the cause was not attributed to low levels of iron in the food, but to a high fat content in the diet which may inhibit iron absorption. Haymes (1972) studied plasma iron levels and total iron binding capacity and found 25 percent of the trained female field hockey players, 32 percent of the moderately active females, and 8 percent of the sedentary females were iron deficient. Clement and others (1977) suggested that the hemoglobin levels of Canadian Olympic athletes were significantly lower than the normal population in Canada, although the values were in the normal range. Ehn and others (1980) reported extremely low bone marrow iron stores in elite distance runners, even though their hemoglobin and serum iron levels were normal. Thus, it appears that some athletes, particularly females, may be iron deficient.

There have been some suggestions that physical conditioning, particularly in the initial stages, may produce a condition known as sports anemia in untrained individuals. Dietary insufficiency of protein and/or iron have been hypothesized as causative factors, and this issue is addressed elsewhere in this symposium. Whether or not an iron deficiency occurs during the early stages of training is controversial. Kilbom (1971) found significant decreases in serum iron during seven weeks of moderate intensity training and similar findings were reported by Haymes (1975) and Gardus and others (1981). However, Fox (Mathews and Fox, 1976) did not confirm these results. In trained athletes, Puhl and Runyan (1980) noted that an increase in training did not produce any signficiant negative changes in any of the iron related blood variables that they studied. On the other hand Radomski and others (1980) reported the development of sports anemia in trained individuals similar to that found in untrained individuals.

Athletes who train in warm or hot environments may need more iron in their diet. The low to zero levels of bone marrow iron in elite distance runners was suggested to be due to excessive loss of iron in sweat during training (Ehn et al, 1980). Studying subjects at rest in a hot environment, Consolazio and others (1963) and Vellar (1968) both reported significant losses of iron in sweat, up to 0.5 mg/hour. During exercise Thapar and others (1976) reported losses of up to 2.5 mg/liter of sweat while Kavanagh and Shephard (1976) recorded losses of 4.5 mg/liter of sweat after a marathon race.

Anemia with low hemoglobin levels would impair oxygen transport and, hence, endurance capacity, and this point has been extensively documented (Anderson and Barkue, 1970; Charlton et al, 1977; Davies and Van Haaren, 1973; Davies et al, 1973; Gardner et al, 1977). It has also been established that iron supplementation to individuals with iron deficiency anemia will increase performance capacity (Davies and Van Haaren, 1973; Edgerton et al, 1979; Gardner et al, 1975; Gardner and Edgerton, 1972; Hermansen, 1973).

Although iron supplementation would be expected to benefit the iron-deficient anemic person, of what value might it be to the athlete? There has been relatively little controlled research done in this area, and yet, based on previous epidemiological studies dealing with iron deficiency, there may be apparent justification for recommending increased iron content in the diet or iron tablets for women athletes. Some authorities have recommended outright iron supplementation. deWijn and his colleagues (1971a; 1971b) suggested that prophylactic iron supplementation during training is indicated in many top athletes, while Mayer and Bullen (1959) recommended iron supplementation for women who lose over 60 ml blood during the menstrual cycle. White (1974) concurs with this latter recommendation. Many oral preparations of iron are available, and the simple ferrous salts such as sulfate and fumarate are the best absorbed and least expensive. Haymes (1973), after reviewing the literature, concluded that coaches should give serious consideration to the iron content in the diet of their female athletes. Buskirk and Haymes (1972), relating to the nutritional needs of the woman in sports, noted there may be a greater need for iron at the beginning of training, probably due to increased synthesis of myoglobin and the cytochromes.

Although the above recommendations may theoretically be valid, there appears to be little objective data to support the value of additional iron, in the form of iron supplement tablets, to the male or female athlete with normal hemoglobin levels. Several Russian studies (Rusin et al, 1976; Vlasenko, 1980) have reported increased serum iron levels in athletes following iron supplementation. They also noted increased performance levels, but the data is confusing. For example, in one of the studies (Rusin et al, 1976) both the placebo and iron group increased their performance significantly. Ericsson (1970) reported significant increases in elderly subjects following iron supplementation, but attributed the results to factors other than hemoglobin changes. On the other hand Weswig and Winkler (1974), Cooter and Mowbray (1978) and Pate and Others (1979) did not find any significant effect of iron supplementation to athletes on such parameters as hemoblobin, hematocrit, RBC, serum iron, or total iron binding capacity. Relative to performance, Davies and Van Haaren (1973) reported no significant effect of 200 mg iron daily for three months on predicted maximal oxygen uptake.

As noted previously (Beutler, 1980; Pate, 1979) it has not been established whether iron deficiency without anemia impairs physical performance. Nilson and others (1981) recently studied the effect of iron supplementation upon endurance capacity, VO_2 max and lactate production in iron-deficient non-anemic athletes and a control group of athletes. Following a pre-test, 300 mg ferrous sulfate was taken every 8 hours for 10-14 days. Although serum iron levels returned to normal in the iron deficient subjects, no improvement in VO_2 max or time to exhaustion occurred. However, blood lactate levels during maximal exercise were lower following supplementation and the authors hypothesized that the iron dependent oxidative reactions in the muscle tissue were enhanced, thus facilitating aerobic metabolism.

Although remote, there may be some danger from prolonged consumption of large amounts of iron. White, Handler and Smith (1973) noted that since there is no excretory pathway for excess iron, it tends to accumulate as hemosiderin in the liver in quantities sufficient to result in ultimate destruction of that organ. Hemochromotosis, characterized by pigmentation of the skin and hepatic cirrhosis, may result from excessive iron salt administration.

As an aside, the technique of blood doping, the infusion of blood into the athlete, may have therapeutic implications for the anemic athlete or those with subnormal levels of hemoglobin. A discussion of blood doping and the relevant research has been presented by Williams (1981a, 1981b).

Calcium

The vast majority, or 99 percent, of calcium is present in the skeleton while 1 percent serves a number of physiological functions unrelated to bone structure. It is required as a component in a number of enzyme systems, particularly in muscle contraction in both the heart and skeletal muscle, nerve impulse transmission and blood clotting. Thus, any major change in calcium balance could be detrimental to bone development or normal nervous and muscular tissue functioning. However, the average individual on a balanced diet will not suffer a calcium deficiency and no case of sufficient severity to affect the health of the nervous system has been recorded (White, 1974). Nevertheless, adequate calcium intake should be assured during the developmental years of youth and adolescence, and calcium supplements have been recommended for older females, as bone mineral content decreases at the rate of one percent/year after age 35 (Smith et al, 1981).

Research is limited relative to calcium supplementation and physical performance, and there are little or no implications that it is necessary. However, requirements may be increased somewhat during exercise in a hot environment. The mean intake of calcium is 400-1300 mg/day. Avioli (1980) notes that the average adult may maintain calcium balance on 600-1000 mg/day, whereas growing children and older adults may need slightly greater amounts. Avioli also noted that calcium losses in sweat may approximate one gram/day in individuals working at high temperatures. Consolazio and others (1962) suggested that calcium requirements are increased under conditions of heavy sweat losses, and stated that it is questionable whether an individual consuming a low calcium diet could attain calcium balance under such conditions. On the other hand, they also noted that the subjects in their study were in calcium balance at 441 mg/day without sweat losses; the sweat losses created a negative balance of 100-150 mg. Hence, an additional dietary source could easily correct this deficiency. Nevertheless, the athlete who exercises regularly in environmental temperatures which elicit profuse sweating should be sure to include calcium rich foods, notably dairy products, in the diet. It should also be noted that acclimitization helps to decrease calcium losses in the sweat.

Calcium supplements may help prevent osteoporosis in inactive elderly females, but exercise may elicit the same effect. Smith and others (1981) studied elderly women (69-95) over a 3 year span investigating the effect of physical activity and calcium (.75 g/day) and vitamin D (400 IU/day) upon bone mineral content (BMC). Subjects were matched and assigned to one of 4 groups: control, supplement, exercise, or exercise and supplement. The results indicated a decrease in BMC of the control group while the other 3 groups increased their BMC. Both exercise and the supplement alone were effective, but there was no additive effect in the group that had both treatments.

Calcium supplementation may be used by some athletes in the form of the so-called vitamin B_{15}, also known as pangamic acid. One form of pangamic acid is calcium pangamate, usually consisting of calcium gluconate and dimethylglycine (DMG). Several investigators have studied the effects of calcium pangamate upon human physical performance. Pipes (1980) reported that 5 mg of pangamic acid for 7 days increased VO_2 max by 27.5 percent and treadmill run time to exhaustion by 23.6 percent. However, few details were presented in this brief abstract and the author did not appear to report his paper at the 1980 meeting of the American College of Sports Medicine. Two other well-controlled studies do not support a beneficial effect of calcium pangamate. Girandola and other (1980) administered 2.5 calcium gluconate and DMG to 8 subjects for 2 weeks. They reported no significant improvements in cardiovascular or metabolic parameters at a work rate of 70 percent VO_2 max. Black and Sucec (1981) tested 18 physically active men via a counterbalanced repeated measures design. Dependent variables were VO_2 max, anaerobic threshold and 15 minute run performance. Three trials were utilized—control, placebo and supplement. The supplement was 300 mg/day of calcium gluconate and DMG. Their results revealed no significant difference between the trails and the authors concluded there was no measurable effect of the prescribed dosage of calcium pangomate.

One should be cautious in the use of vitamin B_{15} compounds as Victor Herbert has noted the term is chemically meaningless so producers can put anything they want into a bottle and label it vitamin B_{15} or pangamic acid; moreover, a component often found in some preparations of vitamin B_{15} has been shown to be mutagenic and may cause cancer (Check, 1980).

Zinc

Zinc is associated with a variety of enzymes including carbonic anhydrose and lactic acid dehydrogenose. Li (1980) has indicated that there is a deficiency syndrome now being recognized in the United States, particularly in young individuals with prolonged intestinal malabsorption. Failure to grow and anorexia are clinical symptoms. A recent report (Dressendorfer and Sockolov, 1980) noted that the serum zinc levels in a number of long distance runners were on the extreme lower level of normal and they were considered to be hypozincemic, presumably due to increased losses of zinc in sweat. Although the runners did have low zinc levels, they experienced no problems. The authors suggested that a low serum zinc level is not conclusive evidence of abnormal zinc status and did not recommend supplements.

Other Trace Elements

Some of the trace elements have functions related to the metabolic processes that are activated during exercise. However, these elements have not been studied as supplements to improve physical performance capacity. Copper is essential to prevent anemia, even in the presence of adequate supplies of iron; copper is also involved in energy metabolism as it is a constituent of cytochrome oxidase (Dowdy, 1969). Cobalt is a constituent of vitamin B_{12}, necessary for prevention of anemia. Chromium is required for maintaining normal glucose metabolism in experimental animals, and may have similar functions in man. Manganese appears to be essential for normal functioning of the central nervous system. Although all of these trace elements and others are important regulators of numerous physiological processes in the body, Mayer and Bullen (1959) noted that a pure or complete deficiency of trace elements in man is obviously unlikely.

SUMMARY

Although the general implications of this review would be that vitamin and mineral supplements are ineffective as ergogenic aids when added to the diet of an athlete who is well-nourished, there may be certain cases where supplementation is warranted. For example, wrestlers on low-calorie diets and high levels of energy expenditure may not be receiving a balanced intake of nutrients. Young male athletes and female athletes of all ages should be aware of iron-rich foods and include them in the daily diet. The female athlete who experiences heavy menstrual flow may consider commercial iron preparations; hemoglobin and other hemotological determinations may be evaluated in order to determine the need for supplementation.

More research is needed, particularly with large doses of the vitamin B complex and vitamin C. Although some of the studies cited herein have used rather large doses, some athletes have been reported to consume rather massive dosages, e.g. 10,000 mg vitamin C daily. Unfortunately, there may be some adverse side effects of such massive doses and it may not be ethical to conduct research with humans at those high intake levels. Do these massive dosages elicit a pharmacodynamic effect on some metabolic reactions favorable to physical performance? More research with vitamin E at altitude also appears warranted, as does iron supplementation to iron-deficient, but not anemic, athletes. As noted above, the current data base suggests that vitamin and mineral supplements are unnecessary for the athlete receiving a balanced diet. However, only with additional controlled research may we expand that data base to help answer some of the questions that still remain relative to nutrition and athletic performance. There are still a large number of athletes who believe that the 'racers edge' may be found in a tablet.

REFERENCES

1. Anderson, H. and Barkue, H. Iron deficiency and muscular work performance. **Scandinavian Journal of Clinical Laboratory Investigation.** 25:Suppl 114, 9-37, 1970.

2. Anonymous. Russians research food requirements of athletes. **Swimming Technique,** 8:59, July, 1971A.

3. Anonymous. Vitamin E in athletics. **British Medical Journal,** 4:251, 1971B.

4. Archdeacon, J. and Murlin, J. The effect of thiamine depletion and restoration on muscular efficiency and endurance. **Journal of Nutrition,** 28:241-54, 1944.

5. Avioli, L. Calcium and phosphorus. In Goodhart, R. and Shils, M. (Eds.) **Modern Nutrition in Health and Disease,** Philadelphia: Lea and Febiger, 1980.

6. Bailey, D. and others. Effect of vitamin C supplementation upon the physiological responses to exercise in trained and untrained runners. **International Zeitschrift Vitaminforch,** 40:435, 1970.

7. Basu, N., and Ray, G. The effect of vitamin C on the incidence of fatigue in human muscles. **Indian Journal of Medical Research,** 28:419-26, 1940.

8. Bentivenga, A., Kelly, E., and Kalenak, A. Diet, fitness and athletic performance. **Physician and Sports Medicine,** 7:00-105, October, 1979.

9. Bergstrom, J., Hultman, E., Jorfeldt, L., Pernow, B., and Wahren, J. Effect of nicotinic acid on physical working capacity and on metabolism of muscle glycogen in man. **Journal of Applied Physiology,** 26:170-76, 1969.

10. Berryman, G. and others. Effects in young men consuming restricted quantities of B complex vitamins and proteins, and changes associated with supplementation. **American Journal of Physiology,** 148:618-47, 1947.

11. Berven, H. The physical working capacity of healthy children. Seasonal variation and effect of ultraviolet radiation and vitamin D supply. **Acta Paediatrica,** 148:Suppl. 1-22, 1963.

12. Beutler, E. Iron. In Goodhart, R. and Shils, M. (Eds.) **Modern Nutrition in Health and Disease.** Philadelphia: Lea and Febiger, 1980.

13. Bialeck, M. Nicotinic acid after physical exertion. **Polski Tygod-nik Lekarski,** 17:1370-1375, 1962.

14. Black, D. and Sucec, A. Effects of calcium pangamate on aerobic endurance parameters. **Medicine and Science of Sports and Exercise,** 13:93, 1981.

15. Bourne, G. Nutrition and Exercise. In Falls, H. (Ed.) **Exercise Physiology,** New York: Academic Press, 1968.

16. Bourne, G. Vitamins and muscular exercise. **British Journal of Nutrition,** 2:261-63, 1948.

17. Brozek, J. Soviet studies on nutrition and higher nervous activity. **Annals New York Academy of Sciences,** 93:667-714, 1962.

18. Buskirk, E. and Haymes, E. Nutritional requirements for women in sport. In Harris, D. (Ed.) **Women and Sport: A National Research Conference.** University Park: Penn State University, 1972.

19. Cardus, D., Ribas-Cardus, F. and McTaggert, W. Changes in blood viscosity with exercise training. **Medicine and Science in Exercise and Sports,** 13:109, 1981.

20. Carlson, L., and Oro, L. The effect of nicotinic acid on the plasma free fatty acids. **Acta Medica Scandinavica,** 172:641-45, 1962.

21. Carlson, L., Havel, R. and Ekelund, L. Effect of nicotinic acid on the turnover rate and oxidation of the free fatty acids of plasma in man during exercise. **Metabolism,** 12:837-45, 1963.

22. Charlton, R., Derman, D., Skikne, B., and others. Anaemia, iron deficiency and exercise: extended studies in human subjects. **Clinical Science and Molecular Medicine,** 53:537-541, 1977.

23. Chase, D. John Walker-World's most watched-over athlete. **The Physician and Sportsmedicine,** 4:89-92, February, 1976.

24. Check, W. Vitamin B_{15}-Whatever it is, it won't help. **Journal of the American Medical Association,** 243:2473-2480, 1980.

25. Clausen, D. The combined effect of aerobic exercise and vitamin E upon cardiorespiratory endurance and measured blood variables. Unpublished masters thesis, University of Wyoming, 1971.

26. Clement, D., Asmundson, B. and Medhurst, C. Hemoglobin values: comparative study of the 1976 Canadian olympic team. **Canadian Medical Association Journal,** 117:614-616, 1977.

27. Consolazio, C., Matoush, L., Nelson, R. and others. Excretion of sodium, potassium, magnesium, and iron in human sweat and the relation of each to balance and requirements. **Journal of Nutrition,** 79:407-415, 1963.

28. Consolazio, C., Matoush, L., Nelson, R., and others. Relationship between calcium in sweat, calcium balance and calcium requirements. **Journal of Nutrition,** 78:78-88, 1962.

29. Cooter, G. and Mowbray, K. Effects of iron supplementation and activity on serum iron depletion and hemoglobin levels in female athletes. **Research Quarterly,** 49:114-118, 1978.

30. Csik, L., and Bencsik, J. Versuche die Wirkung von B-vitamin aud die Arbeitsleistung des Menschen Festzustellen. **Klinische Wochenschrift,** 6:2275-2278, 1927.

31. Cureton, T. The diet of schoolboy athletes can be improved. **Athletic Journal,** 50:71, September, 1969A.

32. Cureton, T. Nutritive aspects of physical fitness work. **Swimming Technique,** 6:44-49, July, 1969B.

33. Cureton, T. Wheat germ oil, the "wonder" fuel. **Scholastic Coach,** 24:36, March, 1955.

34. Davies, C. and Van Haaren, J. Effect of treatment on physiological responses to exercise in East African industrial workers with iron deficiency anemia. **British Journal of Industrial Medicine,** 30: 335-40, 1973.

35. Davies, C. and others. Iron deficiency anemia: its effect on maximum aerobic power and responses to exercise in African males aged 17-40 years. **Clinical Science,** 44:555-62, 1973.

36. Davis, T. and others. Review of studies of vitamin and mineral nutrition in the United States (1950-1968). **Journal of Nutrition Education,** 1:Suppl. 1, 41-45, 1969.

37. deWijn J., and others: Hemoglobin, packed cell volume, serum iron, and iron building capacity of selected athletes during training. **Journal of Sports Medicine and Physical Fitness,** 11:42-51, 1971A.

38. deWijn, J., and others. Hemoglobin, packed cell volume, serum iron, and iron building capacity of selected athletes during training. **Nutrition and Metabolism,** 13:129-39, 1971B.

39. Dowdy, R. Copper Metabolism. **American Journal of Clinical Nutrition,** 22:387-91, 1969.

40. Dressendorfer, R. and Sockolov, R. Hypozincemia in runners. **The Physician and Sportsmedicine,** 8:97-100, April, 1980.

41. Durnin, J. The influence of nutrition. **Canadian Medical Association Journal,** 96:715-20, 1967.

42. Early, R., and Carlson, B. Water soluble vitamin therapy on the delay of fatigue from physical activity in hot climatic conditions. **Internationale Zeitschrfit fur Angewandte Physiologie,** 27:43-50, 1969.

43. Edgerton, V., Gardner, G., Ohira, Y., and others. Iron deficiency anemia and its effect on worker productivity and activity patterns. **British Medical Journal,** 2:1546-1549, Dec 15, 1979.

44. Egana, E. and others. The effects of a diet deficient in the vitamin B complex on sedentary men. **American Journal of Physiology,** 127:731-41, 1942.

45. Ehn, L., Carlmark, B., and Hoglund, S. Iron status in athletes involved in_intense physical activity. **Medicine and Science of Sports and Exercise,** 12:61-64, 1980.

46. Ericsson, P. The effect of iron supplementation on the physical work capacity in the elderly. **Acta Medica Scandinavica,** 188:361-74, 1970.

47. Foltz, E., Ivy, A., and Barborka, C. Influence of components of the vitamin B complex on recovery from fatigue. **Journal of Laboratory and Clinical Medicine,** 27:1396-1399, 1942.

48. Fox, F., Dangerfield, L., Gottlich, S., and Jokl, E. Vitamin C requirements of native workers. **British Medical Journal,** 2:143-47, 1940.

49. Frankau, I. Acceleration of co-ordinated muscular effort by nicotinamide. **British Medical Journal,** 2:601-603, 1943.

50. Gardner, G. and Edgerton, V.R. Iron deficiency and physical work performance. Paper presented at National ACSM Meeting, Philadelphia, May, 1972.

51. Gardner, G. and Edgerton, V., Senewirante, B., and others. Physical work capacity and metabolic stress in subjects with iron deficiency anemia. **American Journal of Clinical Nutrition,** 30:910-917, 1977.

52. Gardner, G. and Edgerton, V., Barnard, R., and others. Cardiorespiratory, hematological, and physical performance responses of anemic subjects to iron treatment. **American Journal of Clinical Nutrition,** 28:982-988, 1975.

53. Gey, G., Cooper, K., and Bottenberg, R. Effects of ascorbic acid on endurance performance and athletic injury. **Journal of the American Medical Association,** 211:105, 1970.

54. Girandola, R., Wiswell, R., and Bulbulian, R. Effects of pangamic acid (B-15) ingestion on metabolic response to exercise. **Medicine and Science of Sports and Exercise,** 12:98, 1980.

55. Gounelle, H. Action de la vitamine B, dans L'exercise musculaire et la prevention de la fatigue. **Bulletin et memoires de la Societe medicale des hopitaux de Paris,** 56:255-57, 1940.

56. Grandjean, A., Hursh, L., Majure, W. and Hanley, D. Nutrition knowledge and practices of college athletes. **Medicine and Science of Sports and Exercise,** 13:82, 1981.

57. Hamilton, E. and Whitney, E. **Nutrition: Concepts and Controversies.** St. Paul: West Publishing Co., 1979.

58. Hanely, D. The catastrophic triviality. **Nutrition Today,** 3:17-20, 1968.

59. Haralambie, G. Vitamin B_2 status in athletes and the influence of riboflavin administration on neuromuscular irritability. **Nutrition and Metabolism,** 20:1-8, 1976.

60. Haralambie, G. and Berg, A. Changes in physiologic and biochemical values following exertion test in women with and without calcium substitution. **Medizin Welt,** 30:1233-1238, 1979.

61. Haymes, E. Iron deficiency and women athletes. Paper presented at the American College of Sports Medicine National Meeting, New Orleans, May, 1975.

62. Haymes, E. Iron deficiency and the active woman. **DGWS Research Reports,** 2:91-7, 1973.

63. Haymes, E. The effect of physical activity level on selected hematological variables in adult women. Paper presented at the National AAHPER Convention. Houston, March, 1972.

64. Henschel, A., Taylor, H., Brozek, J., Mickelsen, O., and Keys, A. Vitamin C and ability to work in hot environments. **American Journal of Tropical Medicine and Hygiene,** 24:259-65, 1944.

65. Herbert, V., Colman, N. and Jacob, E. Folic Acid and vitamin B_{12}. In Goodhart, R. and Shils, M. **Modern Nutrition in Health and Disease,** Philadelphia: Lea and Febiger, 1980.

66. Hermansen, L. Oxygen Transport during exercise in human subjects. **Acta Physiologica Scandinavica Supplement,** 399:9-104, 1973.

67. Hilsendager, D., and Karpovich, P. Ergogenic effect of glycine and niacin separately and in combination. **Research Quarterly,** 35:389-92, 1964.

68. Hirata, I. Pre-game meals: a discussion. **Swimming Technique,** 10:22-24, April, 1973.

69. Hoglund, S., Ehn, L., and Lieden, G. Iron deficiency in young men. **Acta Haematologica,** 44:193-199, 1970.

70. Hoitink, A. Vitamin C and Work. Leiden: **Nederlands Instituut voor Praeventieve Geneeskunde TNO,** 1946A.

71. Hoitink, A. Researches on the influence of vitamin C administration on the human organism, in particular in connection with the working capacity. **Acta Brevia Neerleandicaade Physiologia, Pharmacologia Microbiologia,** 14:62, 1946B.

72. Hoogerwerf, A., and Hoitink, A. The influence of vitamin C administration on the mechanical effiency of the human organism. **Internationale Zeitschrift fur Angewandte Physiologie,** 20:164-72, 1963.

73. Horak, J. and others. Ascorbic acid blood level prior to laboratory work and after: Its relationship to spiroergometric parameters in top-performance athletes. **Casopis Lekaru Ceskych,** 116:679-82, 1977.

74. Horstman, D. Nutrition. In Morgan, W. (Ed.): **Ergogenic Aids and Muscular Performance,** New York: Academic Press, 1972.

75. Horwitt, M. Riboflavin. In Goodhart, R. and Shils, M (Eds.) **Modern Nutrition in Health and Disease.** Philadelphia: Lea and Febiger, 1980.

76. Howald, H. and Segesser, B. Ascorbic acid and athletic performance. **Annals New York Academy of Science,** 258:458, 1975.

77. Jetzler, A., and Haffter, C. Vitamin C-Bedarf bei einmaligar sportlicher Dauerleistung. **Wiener Medizinische Wochenschrift,** 89:332, 1939.

78. Jokl, E., and Suzman, H. A study of the effects of vitamin C upon physical efficiency, **Transvaal Mine Medical Officers Association Proceedings,** 19:292-300, March, 1940

79. Karpovich, P., and Millman, N. Vitamin B and endurance. **New England Journal of Medicine,** 226:881-82, 1942.

80. Kavanagh, T. and Shephard, R. Fluid and mineral balance in post-coronary marathon runners. In Bard, C. and other (Eds.) **Abstracts of the International Congress of Physical Activity Sciences.** Quebec City: CISAP, 1976.

81. Keren, G. The effect of high dosage vitamin C intake on aerobic and anaerobic capacity. **Journal of Sports Medicine and Physical Fitness,** 20:145-8, 1980.

82. Keys, A. Physical performance in relation to diet. **Federal Proceedings,** 2:164-87, 1943.

83. Keys, A. and others. Experimental studies on men with a restricted intake of the B vitamins. **American Journal of Physiology,** 144:5-42, 1945.

84. Keys, A. and others. The performance of normal young men on controlled thiamine intake. **Journal of Nutrition,** 26:399-415, 1943.

85. Kilbom, A. Physical training in women. **Scandinavian Journal of Clinical and Laboratory Investigation,** 28:Suppl: 119, 1971.

86. Kirchoff, H. Uber den Einfluss von Vitamin C auf Energieverbrauch, Kreislauf and Ventilationensgnossen im Belastungversuch. **Nutritio Dieta (Basel),** 11:184, 1969.

87. Klafs, C., and Arnheim, D. **Modern Principles of Athletic Training.** St. Louis, Mosby, 1973.

88. Kobayashi, Y. Effect of vitamin E on aerobic work performance in men during acute exposure to hypoxic hypoxia. Ph.D Dissertation, University of New Mexico, Albuquerque, 1974.

89. Lamb, L. Vitamin C (Ascorbic Acid). **The Health Letter,** 3:1-4, 1974.

90. Lawrence, J., Bower, R., Riehl, W., and Smith, J. Effects of alpha-tocopherol acetate on the swimming endurance of trained swimmers. **American Journal of Clinical Nutrition,** 28:205-208, 1974A.

91. Lawrence, J., Smith, J., Bower, R., and Riehl, W. The effect of alpha-tocopherol (Vitamin E) and Pyridoxine HC1 (Vitamin B_6) on the swimming endurance of trained swimmers. **Journal of the American College Health Association,** 23:219-22, 1974B.

92. Li, T. and Vallee, B. The biochemical and nutritional roles of other trace elements. In Goodhart, R. and Shils, M. (Eds.) **Modern Nutrition in Health and Disease,** Philadelphia: Lea and Fabiger, 1980.

93. Margaria, R., Aghemo, P., and Rovelli, E. The effect of some drugs on the maximal capacity of athletic performance in man. **Internationale Zeithschrift Angewandte Physiologie,** 20:281-87, 1964.

94. Mathews, D. and Fox, E. **The Physiological Basis of Physical Education and Athletics,** Philadelphia: W.B. Saunders, 1976.

95. Mayer, J., and Bullen, B. Nutrition and athletic performance. **Postgraduate Medicine,** 26:848-56, 1959.

96. McCormick, W. Vitamin B and physical endurance. **Medical Record,** 152:439, 1940.

97. Montoye, H. Vitamin B_{12}: A review. **Research Quarterly,** 26:308-13, 1955.

98. Montoye, H., Spata, P., Pinckney, V., and Barron, L. Effects of vitamin B_{12} supplementation on physical fitness and growth of young boys. **Journal of Applied Physiology,** 7:589-92, 1955.

99. Nagawa, T. and others. The effect of Vitamin E on endurance. **Asian Medical Journal,** 11:619-33, 1968.

100. Namyslowski, L. Observations concerning the influence of Vitamin C on the physical fitness of sportsmen. **Sportartzliche Praxis,** 3:118-19, 1960.

101. National Research Council: Committee on Dietary Allowances: **Recommended Dietary Allowances.** Washington: National Academy of Sciences, 1974.

102. Nijakowski, F. Assays of some vitamins of the B complex group in human blood in relation to muscular effort. **Acta Physiologica Polonica,** 17:Suppl, 397-404, 1966.

103. Nilson, K., Schone, R., Robertson, H., and others. The effect of iron repletion on exercise-induced lactate production in minimally iron-depleted subjects. **Medicine and Science of Sports and Exercise,** 13:92, 1981.

104. Nocker, J. Nutrition and performance. **Internist,** 11:269-73, 1970.

105. Novich, M. Drug abuse and drugs in sport. **New York State Journal of Medicine,** 73:2597-2600, 1973.

106. Pate, R., Maguire, M., and Van Wyk, J. Dietary iron supplementation in women athletes. **The Physician and Sports Medicine,** 7:81-88, Sept., 1979.

107. Percival, L. Vitamin E in athletic efficiency. Shute Foundation for Medical Research, December, 1951, 3, No.2.

108. Peterson, C. Problems of iron imbalance. **Drug Therapy,** (Hosp): 61-74, February, 1979.

109. Pipes, T. The effects of pangamic acid on performance in trained athletes. **Medicine and Science of Sports and Exercise,** 12:98, 1980.

110. Potenza, P. Estere fosforico della riboflavina et fatica. **Vitaminologia,** 17:345-350, 1959.

111. Puhl, J. and Runyan, W. Hematology of women cross-country runners during training. **Medicine and Science of Sports and Exercise,** 12:108, 1980.

112. Radomski, M., Sabiston, B. and Isoard, P. Development of "Sports anemia" in physically fit men after daily sustained submaximal exercise. **Aviation and Space Environmental Medicine,** 51:41-45, 1980.

113. Rasch, P., Arnheim, D., and Klafs, C. Effects of vitamin C supplementation on cross-country runners. **Sportartzliche Praxis,** 5:10-13, Heft I, 1962.

114. Richardson, J., Palmerton, T., and Chenan, M. The effect of calcium on muscle fatigue. **Journal of Sports Medicine and Physical Fitness,** 20:149-51, 1980.

115. Rusin, V., Nasolodin, V. and Vorobyov, V. Iron, copper, manganese and zinc metabolism in athletes under high physical pressures. **Voprosy Pitaniia,** (4): 15-19,1980.

116. Rusin, V. and others. On the analysis of iron allowance in the organism of sportswomen-skiers. **Voprosy Pitaniia,** (6):65-9, 1976.

117. Ryan, A. Nutritional Practices in athletics abroad. **The Physician and Sportsmedicine,** 5:33-44, January, 1977.

118. Sakaeva, E., and Efremov, V. Experience with additional allowance of vitamin E to sportsmen-race cyclists and skiers. **Vestnik Akademii Meditsinskikh Nauk SSSR,** 27:52-55, 1972.

119. Seidl, E. and Hettinger, T. Der Einfluss von Vitamin D_3 auf Kraft und Leistungs-fahigkeit des gesunden Erwachsenen. **Internationale Zeitschrift fur Angewandte Physiologie,** 16:365-72, 1957.

120. Sharman, I. and others. The effect of vitamin E on physiological function and athletic performance on trained swimmers. **Journal of Sports Medicine and Physical Fitness,** 16:215-25, 1976.

121. Sharman, I. The effects of vitamin E and training on physiological function and athletic performance in adolescent swimmers. **British Journal of Nutrition,** 26:265-76, 1971.

122. Shephard, R., Campbell, R., Pimm, P., Stuart, D., and Wright, G. Do athletes need Vitamin E. **The Physician and Sportsmedicine,** 2:57-60, September, 1974A.

123. Shephard, R., Campbell, R., Pimm, P., Stuart, D., and Wright, G. Vitamin E, exercise, and the recovery from physical activity. **European Journal of Applied Physiology,** 33:119-126, 1974B.

124. Sherman, H. and Smith, S. **The Vitamins.** New York: The Chemical Catalogue Co., 1922.

125. Simonson, E., Enzer, N., Baer, A., and Braun, R. The influence of vitamin B (complex) surplus on the capacity for muscular and mental work. **Journal of Industrial Hygiene,** 24:83-90, 1942.

126. Smith, E., Reddan, W., and Smith, P. Physical activity and calcium modalities for bone mineral increase in aged women. **Medicine and Science of Sports and Exercise,** 13:60-64, 1981.

127. Spioch, F., Kobza, R., and Mazur, B. Influence of vitamin C upon certain functional changes and the coefficient of mechanical efficiency in humans during physical effort, **Acta Physiologica Polonica,** 17:251-64, 1966.

128. Stewart, G. and others. Observations on the haemotology and the iron and protein intake of Australian olympic athletes. **Medical Journal of Australia,** 2:1339-43, 1972.

129. Talbot, D. Vitamin supplements are essential. **Sport and Fitness Instructor,** June, 1974.

130. Thapar, G., Shenolikar, I. and Tulpule, P. Sweat loss of nitrogen and other nutrients during heavy physical activity. **Indian Journal of Medical Research,** 64:590-596, 1976.

131. Tin-May-Than, Ma-Win-May, Khin-Sann-Aung, and M. Mya-Tu. The effect of vitamin B_{12} on physical performance capacity. **British Journal of Nutrition,** 40:269-73, 1978.

132. United States Senate. **Proper and improper use of drugs by athletes.** (Hearings before the subcommittee to investigate juvenile delinquency, June 18 and July 12-13, 1973). Washington, D.C.: U.S. Government Printing Office, 1973.

133. Van Huss, W. What made the Russians run? **Nutrition Today,** 1:20-23, 1966.

134. Van Huss, W. Vitamins and performance with emphasis on Vitamin C. National American College of Sports Medicine meeting, Knoxville, Tennessee, May 9, 1974.

135. Vellar, O. Studies on sweat losses of nutrients: I. Iron content of whole body sweat and its association with other sweat constituents, serum iron levels, hematological indices, body surface area and sweat rate. **Scandinavian Journal of Clinical Investigation,** 21:157-167, 1968.

136. Vlasenko, K. Effect of biotic doses of manganese and hemostimulin on the physical work capacity of athletes 13 to 16 years old. **Voprosy Pitaniia,** (4):19-22, 1980.

137. Vtchikova, M. Increasing the vitamin B_1 content in the rations of athletes. **Chemical Abstracts,** 52:14787, 1958.

138. Wald, G., Brouha, L., and Johnson, R. Experimental human vitamin A deficiency and ability to perform muscular exercise. **American Journal of Physiology,** 137:551-56, 1942.

139. Watt, T., McGuey, D. Allen, C., Goode, R., Romet, T., and McFarlane, I. Letter: Vitamin E and oxygen consumption. **Lancet,** 2:354-55, August 10, 1974.

140. Weswig, P. and Winkler, W. Iron supplementation and hematological data of competition swimmers. **Journal of Sports Medicine and Physical Fitness,** 14:112-19, 1974.

141. White, A., Handler, P., and Smith, E. **Principles of Biochemistry.** New York: McGraw-Hill, 1973.

142. White, P.: **Let's talk about food.** Acton, Massachusetts: Publishing Sciences Group, 1974.

143. Williams, M. Blood Doping: An update. **The Physician and Sports-medicine,** 9:59-63, July, 1981.

144. Williams, M. Blood Doping in Sports. **Journal of Drug Issues,** 10:331-39, 1980.

145. Wolf, E., Wirth, J. and Lohman, T. Nutritional practices of coaches in the Big Ten. **The Physician and Sportsmedicine,** 7:113-124, February, 1979.

146. Yakovlev, N. and Rogozkin, V. Sports biochemistry in the Soviet Union. Paper presented at the National American College of Sports Medicine meeting. New Orleans, May, 1975.

Summary

Dr. Williams' extensive review of the influence of vitamin and mineral supplementation on athletic performance emphasized the general lack of definitive studies in this very important area. However, a number of issues were raised that warrant discussion.

It was pointed out by various symposium participants that the diets of athletes probably are no better balanced than those of the general population. But, since the training athlete consumes more energy than the average individual, he probably makes up in volume for any nutrient shortages that would otherwise exist. For example, the typical diet supplies about 6 mg. iron per 1000 Kilocalories, which results in an iron intake less than the RDA for an average man or woman who consumes less than 2000 Kilocalories per day. But it is not for the athlete who consumes 3000 or more Kilocarloies per day (who would be obtaining the USRDA of 18 mg. of iron). Therefore, the increase in caloric turnover protects the athlete to some extent.

However, this protection of the athletes would probably not hold true for certain athletes, such as ballet dancers or women gymnasts, where weight consciousness is of supreme concern. In fact, women, in general, due to social pressures to be trim, are less prone to meet the RDA for iron.

There was consideration of the lack of well-designed studies of the impact of moderate vitamin and mineral deficiences on athletic performance. Those studies that have been conducted suggest that a major or serious deficiency will show up in reduced performance before it would produce clinical manifestations of a deficiency. These data support the contention that it is important for athletes to maintain the RDA of all nutrients to insure optimal performance. Where there is any doubt about the adequacy of the vitamin and mineral intake of athletes, it would seem appropriate to use some modest form of supplementation (e.g., 1/4 RDA) as a means of insurance.

This led to a discussion of the importance of discriminating between mega-vitamin or mega-mineral supplementation, and such modest supplementation to insure that RDA requirements are met, especially in the growing young athlete. That is, the degree of supplementation that may be of value needs to be considered, not just whether or not to supplement.

An interesting question was raised regarding emphasis on performance criteria to determine the nutritional adequacy of athletes' diets. While performance is certainly one criterion, the long-term health effects of a nutritionally inadequate diet may be more important. Unfortunately, almost nothing is known about the long-term health effects of minor nutrient deficiencies in young or adult athletes. Thus, it may be wrong to look only for changes in athletic performance in response to vitamin or mineral deficiencies or supplementation: the health and quality of life may be the ultimately important criteria.

These later issues led to a discussion of the need for continued long-term surveillance of the eating habits and health status of athletes, not only during training but after they have completed competition as well. Even though endurance athletes who remain active experience less cardiovascular disease than inactive adults, we do not know if other seemingly minor health problems exist. It is important to know if any such problems have a nutritional component.

BODY WEIGHT AND COMPOSITION

Body Composition and Athletic Performance

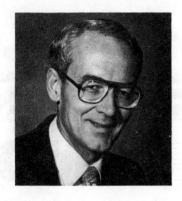

JACK H. WILMORE, PH.D.

Professor, Department of Physical Education, University of Arizona. Member Medical Advisory Board, and former executive director, National Athletic Health Institute. Author of numerous books, chapters, and papers on sports medicine and physiology. Consultant to professional football, basketball and baseball teams, and to President's Council on Physical Fitness and Sports.

How important is one's weight relative to his or her athletic performance? It is not uncommon to read of professional athletes who have been fined rather large sums of money for reporting to training camp "overweight." In many instances the player is fined a certain amount each day for every pound above his or her "desired weight." In some situations, the athlete is told that his bonus, or his salary for the next season, is dependent on his attaining a certain desirable playing weight. One athlete, an all-star major league baseball player, was told that he would receive the $75,000 increase in salary he was asking for, but only if he first lost 25 pounds! At $3,000 per pound, most athletes would be willing to shed quite a few pounds. Fortunately for this athlete, he refused this offer, and on arbitration it was found that he only had 8 pounds of fat, most of which would be considered necessary for his survival!

From the above, two key concepts emerge. First, weight is, and has traditionally been considered important relative to the performance of the athlete. In certain sports such as horse racing, wrestling and boxing, this is obvious. The jockey, wrestler and boxer have certain weights they must attain or they are either penalized or not allowed to compete. In other sports, the coach, trainer or physician either subjectively or objectively determine a weight which they consider to be "ideal" for each of their athletes. It is assumed that any weight above this ideal weight is fat, and is of no value to the athlete. Several studies have found a high, negative relationship between performance in various activities and the relative amount of body fat[1, 6]. The higher the percentage of body fat, the poorer the performance of the individual. This was true of all activities in which the body weight had to be moved either vertically or horizontally through space, e.g. sprinting and long jumping. Many athletes are under the impression that they must be big to be good in their sport. Size has been associated with the quality of the athlete's performance; the bigger the athlete, the better the performance. It is now recognized that this is true only if the size increase is due to an increase in the lean weight of the athlete, i.e. muscle. To add additional fat to the body just to increase overall size is detrimental to performance, with the possible exception of the Sumo wrestler.

The second concept concerns the assumption that every athlete has an "ideal" weight for optimal competition, and that the athlete who exceeds this ideal weight is overweight. While most accept this assumption in theory, there has traditionally been a problem of accurately determining ideal weight and overweight. Overweight is defined as exceeding the maximum weight listed by sex, height, and frame size, from a table of standard values. Unfortunately, these standard tables represent only average or normative data for the population as a whole and don't take into consideration the composition of the body. There are many individuals who are overweight on the basis of the standard height-weight tables, yet who have a normal or lower than normal amount of body fat. Thus, they are overweight by the standard definition, but not overfat. Many athletes tend to fall into this category as a result of their heavy bone structure and large muscle mass.

It is now apparent that our concern must be in evaluating the degree to which the athlete is overfat, and we should not be overly concerned with the athlete who is overweight. In one study of 180 professional football players[7], with an average height of six feet, two inches the standard height weight tables estimated that their average weight should not exceed 194 pounds. Their actual average weight was 220 pounds, or some 26 pounds overweight! When their body fat was assessed by body composition analysis, these athletes were found to have only 13.5% of their total weight as fat, a value which is considerably below the average for their age. They were overweight, but not overfat. The coach, trainer, and physician are thus confronted with the problem of identifying a more valid and objective means of determining competitive weights for their athletes. The remainder of this paper will discuss various techniques for assessing body composition, and will then present data from numerous studies illustrating body composition values for athletes in different sports.

BODY COMPOSITION ASSESSMENT

For purposes of simplicity and convenience of discussion, the total body weight is divided into two components: the lean weight and the fat weight. When working with body composition data, the following relationships are important.

Total body weight = lean body weight + fat weight

Relative body fat = (fat weight/total body weight) × 100

Lean body weight refers to that part of the total body weight which remains after all of the body fat is removed. It is composed of muscle, skin, bone, organs, and all other nonfat tissue. It can be assessed in a number of ways, but the most common is through densitometry, using the underwater weighing technique. The individual is weighed while totally submerged under water after he or she has exhaled all of the air out of the lungs. This weight is then corrected for the buoyancy effect of additional air trapped in the lungs, and pockets of gas in the stomach and intestines.

Archimedes discovered several thousand years ago that the volume of an object can be determined by its loss of weight in water, i.e. actual weight - weight under water. Knowing the volume of a body and its mass or weight, it is possible to calculate the density of that body, since,

$$density = mass/volume.$$

How does this relate to body composition? The density of pure fat is known, and is substantially less than the density of water; thus it will float on water. The density of the lean tissue has been estimated from limited studies on cadavers, and is substantially above that of water. In simple terms, the fat individual will have a low body density and will float with ease in a swimming pool. The lean individual with small amounts of body fat will have a high body density, and will find it difficult, if not impossible, to float. As a second illustration, taking two men of exactly the same height and weight, where one is very fat and the other very lean, when weighed under water the fat individual will weigh considerably less even though the actual weights of the two individuals are identical (Figure 1).

From body density, equations have been established which allow the estimation of relative body fat, i.e. that percentage of the body weight which is fat. From the estimated relative body fat, fat weight and lean body weight can be determined. As an example, an individual who weighs 200 pounds and is found to be 20 percent fat, would have 40 pounds of fat weight (200 pounds × 0.20), and 160 pounds of lean body weight (200 pounds - 40 pounds of fat).

While the body density technique is considered to be the best, or most accurate of the laboratory techniques, it is not without its limitations. Providing the underwater weighing and trapped air volume measurements are conducted properly, the resulting calculation of body density will be accurate. Potential problems exist, however, in the estimation of relative body fat from body density. The equations which have been developed must assume a constant density for both fat and

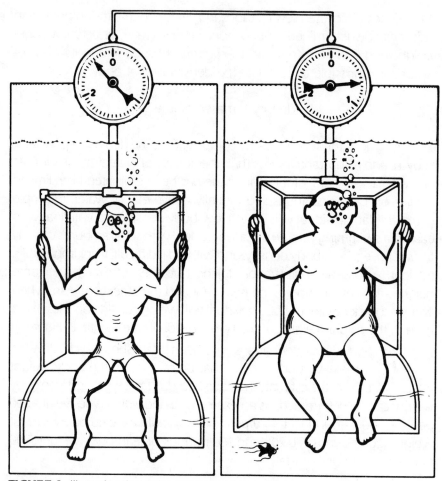

FIGURE 1. *Illustrating the underwater weight technique on two athletes with identical ages, heights and weights, but differing body compositions. Steve is on the left and Tom on the right. Refer to Table 1 for the body composition data.*

lean tissue. The density of fat is relatively consistant from site to site within the body, and from one individual to the next, i.e. 0.900 to 0.907. The density of the lean tissue, however, is quite variable for two reasons. First, the lean tissue is composed of more than one component, e.g. muscle, bone, skin, organs, and it is therefore necessary to estimate the relative contributions of each component to the total lean tissue. If bone is estimated to constitute 23 percent of the lean body mass on the average, a substantial error will occur for the individual whose lean body mass is composed of only 18 percent bone, or the individual whose lean body mass is composed of 27 percent bone. Second, it is assumed that density of each of the components of the lean tissue is constant, when, in fact, there can be considerable variability both within an individual and between individuals. The sum of the variability in proportionality and density of the components of the lean tissue can lead to considerable error, sometimes resulting in negative percentage body fats.

Table 1 illustrates the concepts of body composition discussed to this point, using two athletes of exactly the same age, height, weight, and who are competing for the position of middle linebacker on the university football team. From this assessment it is noted that for an ideal body fat content of 10 percent, Steve is within a pound of his ideal weight while Tom is almost 20 pounds above his ideal. Steve's lean weight is also 16.3 pounds greater, which could be a major factor in determining which of these two individuals wins the starting spot.

While the underwater weighing technique is basically a laboratory technique, it can also be used as a field test. While it is important to determine the residual lung volume in the laboratory setting, to correct the underwater weight for the buoyancy of the trapped air, this value can be estimated in individuals 30 years of age and younger without sacrificing too much accuracy. Estimated residual volumes by age and sex are provided in Table 2.

The underwater weighing can be conducted in a pool, with the scale hung from the diving board or some other form of support. The water should be at least 3 ft deep. The scale should be accurately calibrated prior to use by hanging known weights from it and noting the readings. Since the residual lung volume is measured in liters, weight must also be

TABLE 1. An illustration of the body composition assessment of two athletes of the same age, height, and weight.

Variable	Individual Data			
	Steve		**Tom**	
Height	74.0 in	188.0 cm	74.0 in	188.0 cm
Weight	205.0 lb	93.0 kg	205.0 lb	93.0 kg
Underwater weight (corrected for trapped air)		6.5 kg		5.0 kg
Volume (weight - underwater weight)		86.5 kg		88.0 kg
Density (weight/volume)		1.075 gm/ml		1.057 gm/ml
Relative Fat (495/Density - 450)		10.5%		18.4%
Fat Weight	21.4 lb	9.7 kg	37.7 lb	17.1 kg
Lean Weight	183.6 lb	83.3 kg	167.3 lb	75.9 kg
Weight at 10% fat	204.2 lb	92.6 kg	185.9 lb	84.3 kg
Weight Loss to achieve 10% fat	0.8 lb	0.4 kg	19.1 lb	8.7 kg

TABLE 2. Estimated Residual Lung Volumes by Sex and Age.

Age, Year	Estimated Residual Volume, liters
Females	
6-10	0.60
11-15	0.80
16-20	1.00
21-25	1.20
26-30	1.40
Males	
6-10	0.9
11-15	1.10
16-20	1.30
21-25	1.50
26-30	1.70

'Residual volume also varies with body size; the larger the individual the larger the residual volume. This is partially accounted for by the age corrections up to maturity.

expressed in metric units, i.e. kilograms (weight in pounds divided by 2.205). The individual to be assessed sits on a chair, a weight, or some other type of seat arrangement suspended from the scale, or simply hangs from a rope or chain attached to the scale. The underwater weight of the individual is determined by having him totally submerge, exhaling as much air as possible. The highest weight attained at the conclusion of this maximal exhalation represents the gross underwater weight. A minimum of five to ten trials should be given each individual since it takes practice and experience before an accurate weight can be obtained. The average of the two or three heaviest weights is selected as the representative gross weight for the individual. The weight of the seat, chair, or other supporting material must then be subtracted from the gross weight in order to obtain the individual's actual, or net, weight underwater. Then,

$$\text{Density} = \frac{\text{weight}}{(\text{weight-net underwater weight}) - \text{residual volume}}$$

$$\text{and, Relative Fat (\%)} = (495/\text{Density}) - 450$$

$$\text{Fat Weight (kg)} = \text{Weight} \times \text{Relative Fat}/100$$

$$\text{Lean Weight (kg)} = \text{Weight} - \text{Fat Weight}$$

Technically, the volume of the body should be divided by the density of water corrected for the temperature of the water at the time of the underwater weighing. However, this can be ignored as the values are corrected by less than 1.0 percent.

As an example of the above body composition assessment, an 18 year old male weighs 180 pounds (81.6 kg) and has a net underwater weight of 8 pounds (3.6 kg). From Table 1, the estimated residual volume would be 1.30 liters, and his composition would be as follows:

$$\text{Density} = \frac{81.6}{(81.6-3.6) - 1.30} = \frac{81.6}{76.7} = 1.064$$

Relative Fat (%) = (495/1.064) - 450 = 465.3 - 450 = 15.3%

Fat Weight (kg) = 180 pounds × 15.3%/100 = 27.5 pounds

Lean Weight (kg) = 180 pounds - 27.5 pounds = 152.5 pounds

Assuming the lean weight doesn't change, the individual's weight at any specific percentage of body fat can be determined by dividing the lean weight by the fraction of the total weight that is desired to be lean. To continue the above example, at 10% fat, or 90% lean, the individual would weigh 169.4 pounds, i.e. 152.5 pounds/0.90.

While the hydrostatic or underwater weighing technique is probably the most accurate of the techniques for assessing body composition, it is possible to obtain a reasonably accurate estimate of body composition through anthropometric measurements. Skinfold fat thicknesses, body diameters or breadths, and body circumferences or girths have been used in the past to estimate body density, lean body weight, fat weight, and relative body fat. For purposes of simplification, Table 3 presents equations for males and females of different ages in which density is predicted from skinfolds. For the younger ages, there is a problem in converting the body density to relative body fat, since the individual who has not attained full maturity will have a density of lean tissue which is below that assumed in the equation. This will result in an overestimate of relative body fat. For boys below 18 years of age, and girls below 16 years of age, it may be

TABLE 3. Equations for the prediction of body density from skinfolds in males and females of various ages.

Females

9-12	Density = 1.079 - (0.043 x log of scapula SF)	Parizkova (4)
13-16	Density = 1.102 - (0.058 x log of scapula SF)	Parizkova (4)
17 and above	Density = 1.214 - (0.04057 x log of sum of SF[1]) - (0.00016 x age)	Jackson, Pollock, and Ward (3)

Males

9-12	Density = - 1.054 x log of scapula SF)	Parizkova (4)
13-16	Density = 1.131 - (0.083 x log of triceps SF)	Parizkova (4)
17 and above	Density = 1.189 - (0.0305 x log of sum of SF[2]) - (0.00027 x age)	Jackson and Pollock (2)

[1]Sum of the triceps, suprailiac and thigh skifolds.
[2]Sum of the chest, abdomen and thigh skinfolds.
Note: Take the log of the skinfold, or the sum of the three skinfolds, and multiply it by the designated constant.

advisable to work in density units, which are accurate, and not convert the density value to a percentage of body fat. For males 18 years and older, and females 16 years and older, it is appropriate to convert body density to a percentage body fat.

The anatomical landmarks for the various sites used in the equations in Table 3 are illustrated in Figures 2 through 7. In addition, they are described as follows:

■ **Triceps.** Midway between the acromion and olecranon processes on the posterior aspect of the arm, the arm held vertically, with the fold running parallel to the length of the arm.

■ **Scapula.** Inferior angle of the scapula with the fold running parallel to the vertebral border.

■ **Chest.** Over the lateral border of the pectoralis major, just medial to the axilla, with the fold running diagonally between the shoulder and the opposite hip.

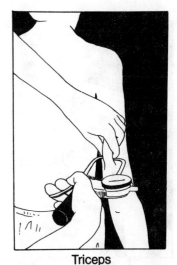

Triceps

FIGURE 2. Illustrating the triceps skinfold site.

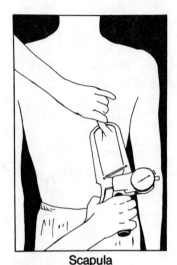

Scapula

FIGURE 3. *Illustrating the scapula skinfold site.*

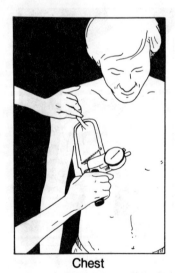

Chest

FIGURE 4. *Illustrating the chest skinfold site.*

■ **Suprailiac.** On the crest of the ilium at the midaxillary line, with the fold running vertically.

■ **Abdomen.** Horizontal fold adjacent to the umbilicus.

■ **Thigh.** Vertical fold on the anterior aspect of the thigh midway between the hip and knee joints.

A special caliper is used to assess the fat that lies directly beneath the skin. The skinfold is grasped firmly by the thumb and index finger, and the caliper is placed on the exact site, approximately one inch from the thumb and finger.

BODY COMPOSITION OF SELECTED ATHLETIC POPULATIONS

Body composition values tend to vary with the sport. Those sports or activities that have a high endurance component, or a strict weight classification system, will typically have athletes characterized by low relative body fats. Long distance runners generally have less than 10 percent body fat. In contrast, males and females of college age will average 13 to 16, and 22-25 percent fat respectively.

Relative body fats for various sports are presented in Table 4. These are not presented as ideal values or goals that the athlete should strive for, since some of these values for both individual and team sports are higher than would normally be considered desirable. For almost all sports, low relative body fats are desirable due to the high negative relationship between performance and percentage body fat as discussed earlier.

From Table 4, it is apparent that the female athlete is typically fatter than her male counterpart, a fact which should not be surprising considering the additional sex-specific fat, e.g. breasts and hips, carried by the female. However, the highly competitive female athlete can attain very low values for relative body fat as illustrated in Figure 8. This figure presents

BODY COMPOSITION AND ATHLETIC PERFORMANCE

relative body fat values for a number of national and international class track and field athletes of various ages. This figure illustrates several important points. First, the better runners generally have low relative body fat values, usually below 12 percent body fat. However, one of the best runners, who held most of the American middle-distance records, was in excess of 17 percent body fat. She was training very intensly, with both high volume and high intensity training. It is unlikely that this athlete could have reduced her relative body fat to levels below 12 percent body fat without having a negative influence on her subsequent performance. This points to the importance of treating each athlete as an individual, and not going strictly by some arbitrarily established guideline. It is appropriate to establish guidelines for each sport or event, e.g. female distance runners should be less than 12 percent fat, but consideration should be given to the exceptions.

The second point illustrated in Figure 8 relates to the high body fat percentages for the discus throwers and shot putters. This figure could leave one with the impression that to be a national-caliber shot putter or discus thrower you need to be fat, i.e. greater than 30 percent body fat. This is quite misleading. First, many of these females were shot put and discus athletes because of their size, not because of their high level of body fat. Most people associate strength and power with body size, so the bigger the athlete the better. One of these shot putters, who went on to shatter the American record, lost a considerable amount of body fat and gained lean body weight through a combination weight training and dietary program. As she continued to lose fat and gain lean weight, her performance continued to improve.

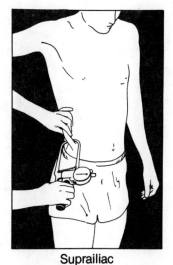

Suprailiac

FIGURE 5. *Illustrating the suprailiac skinfold site.*

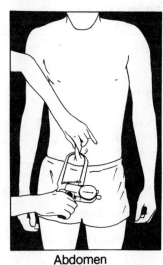

Abdomen

FIGURE 6. *Illustrating the abdomen skinfold site.*

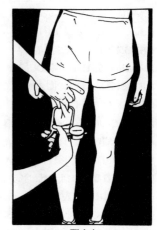

Thigh

FIGURE 7. Illustrating the thigh skinfold site.

TABLE 4. Body Composition Values for Male and Female Athletes.

Athletic Group or Sport	Sex	Age, yr	Height, cm	Weight, kg	Relative Fat, %	Reference
Baseball	male	20.8	182.7	83.3	14.2	Novak, et al
	male	—	—	—	11.8	Forsyth, Sinning
	male[2]	27.4	183.1	88.0	12.6	Wilmore
Basketball	female	19.1	169.1	62.6	20.8	Sinning
	female	19.4	167.0	63.9	26.9	Conger, Macnab
Centers	male[2]	27.7	214.0	109.2	7.1	Parr, et al
Forwards	male[2]	25.3	200.6	96.9	9.0	Parr, et al
Guards	male[2]	25.2	188.0	83.6	10.6	Parr, et al
Canoeing	male	23.7	182.0	79.6	12.4	Rusko, et al
Football	male	20.3	184.9	96.4	13.8	Novak, et al
	male	—	—	—	13.9	Forsyth, Sinning
Defensive Backs	male	17-23	178.3	77.3	11.5	Wickkiser, Kelly
	male[2]	24.5	182.5	84.8	9.6	Wilmore, et al
Offensive Backs	male	17-23	179.7	79.8	12.4	Wickkiser, Kelly
	male[2]	24.7	183.8	90.7	9.4	Wilmore, et al
Linebackers	male	17-23	180.1	87.2	13.4	Wickkiser, Kelly
	male[2]	24.2	188.6	102.2	14.0	Wilmore, et al
Offensive Lineman	male	17-23	186.0	99.2	19.1	Wickkiser, Kelly
	male[2]	24.7	193.0	112.6	15.6	Wilmore, et al

(continued).

TABLE 4. (continued).

Athletic Group or Sport	Sex	Age, yr	Height, cm	Weight, kg	Relative Fat, %	Reference
Defensive Linemen	male	17-23	186.6	97.8	18.5	Wickkiser, Kelly
	male[2]	25.7	192.4	117.1	18.2	Wilmore, et al
Quarterbacks, Kickers	male[2]	24.1	185.0	90.1	14.4	Wilmore, et al
Gymnastics	male	20.3	178.5	69.2	4.6	Novak, et al
	female	19.4	163.0	57.9	23.8	Conger, Macnab
	female	20.0	158.5	51.5	15.5	Sinning, Lindberg
	female	14.0	—	—	17.0	Parizkova
	female	23.0	—	—	11.0	Parizkova
	female	23.0	—	—	9.6	Parizkova
Ice Hockey	male	26.3	180.3	86.7	15.1	Wilmore
	male[2]	22.5	179.0	77.3	13.0	Rusko, et al
Jockeys	male[2]	30.9	158.2	50.3	14.1	Wilmore
Orienteering	male	31.2	—	72.2	16.3	Knowlton, et at
	female	29.0	—	58.1	18.7	Knowlton, et al
Pentathalon	female	21.5	175.4	65.4	11.0	Krahenbuhl, et al
Racketball	male[2]	25.0	181.7	80.3	8.1	Pipes
Rowing						
Heavyweight	male	23.0	192.0	88.0	11.0	Hagerman, et al
Lightweight	male	21.0	186.0	71.0	8.5	Hagerman, et al
	female	23.0	173.0	68.0	14.0	Hagerman, et al
Skiing	male	25.9	176.6	74.8	7.4	Sprynarova, et al
Alpine	male	21.2	176.0	70.1	14.1	Rusko, et al
	male	21.8	177.8	75.5	10.2	Haymes, Dickinson
	female	19.5	165.1	58.8	20.6	Haymes, Dickinson
Cross-Country	male	21.2	176.0	66.6	12.5	Niinimaa, et al
	male	25.6	174.0	69.3	10.2	Rusko, et al
	male	22.7	176.2	73.2	7.9	Haymes, Dickson
	female	24.3	163.0	59.1	21.8	Rusko, et al
	female	20.2	163.4	55.9	15.7	Haymes, Dickson
Nordic Combination	male	22.9	176.0	70.4	11.2	Rusko, et al
	male	21.7	181.7	70.4	8.9	Haymes, Dickson
Skijumping	male	22.2	174.0	69.9	14.3	Rusko, et al
Soccer	male[2]	26.0	176.0	75.5	9.6	Raven, et al
Speed Skating	male	21.0	181.0	76.5	11.4	Rusko, et al

TABLE 4. (continued).

Athletic Group or Sport	Sex	Age, yr	Height, cm	Weight, kg	Relative Fat, %	Reference
Swimming	male	21.8	182.3	79.1	8.5	Sprynarova, et al
	male	20.6	182.9	78.9	5.0	Novak, et al
	female	19.4	168.0	63.8	26.3	Conger, Macnab
Sprint	female	—	165.1	57.1	14.6	Wilmore, et al
Middle-distance	female	—	166.6	66.8	24.1	Wilmore, et al
Distance	female	—	166.3	60.9	17.1	Wilmore, et al
Tennis	male	—	—	—	15.2	Forsyth, Sinning
	male	42.0	179.6	77.1	16.3	Vodak, et al
	female	39.0	163.3	55.7	20.3	Vodak, et al
Track and Field	male	21.3	180.6	71.6	3.7	Novak, et al
	male	—	—	—	8.8	Forsyth, Sinning
Runners	male	22.5	17.4	64.5	6.3	Sprynarova, et al
Distance	male	26.1	175.7	64.2	7.5	Costill, et al
	male	26.2	177.0	66.2	8.4	Rusko, et al
	male	40-49	180.7	71.6	11.2	Pollock, et al
	male	55.3	174.5	63.4	18.0	Barnard, et al
	male	50-59	174.7	67.2	10.9	Pollock, et al
	male	60-69	175.7	67.1	11.3	Pollock, et al
	male	70-75	175.6	66.8	13.6	Pollock, et al
	male	47.2	176.5	70.7	13.2	Lewis, et al
	female	19.9	161.3	52.9	19.2	Malina, et al
	female	32.4	169.4	57.2	15.2	Wilmore, Brown
Middle-Distance	male	24.6	179.0	72.3	12.4	Rusko, et al
Sprint	female	20.1	164.9	56.7	19.3	Malina, et al
	male	46.5	177.0	74.1	16.5	Barnard, et al
Discus	male	28.3	186.1	104.7	16.4	Fahey, et al
	male	26.4	190.8	110.5	16.3	Wilmore
	female	21.1	168.1	71.0	25.0	Malina, et al
Jumpers/Hurdlers	female	20.3	165.9	59.0	20.7	Malina, et al
Shot Put	male	27.0	188.2	112.5	16.5	Fahey, et al
	male	22.0	191.6	126.2	19.6	Behnke, Wilmore
	female	21.5	167.6	78.1	28.0	Malina, et al
Volleyball	female	19.4	166.0	59.8	25.3	Conger, Macnab
	female	19.9	172.2	64.1	21.3	Kovaleski, et al
Weight Lifting	male	24.9	166.4	77.2	9.8	Sprynarova, et al
Power	male	26.3	176.1	92.0	15.6	Fahey, et al

TABLE 4. (continued).

Athletic Group or Sport	Sex	Age, yr	Height, cm	Weight, kg	Relative Fat, %	Reference
Olympic	male	25.3	177.1	88.2	12.2	Fahey, et al
Body Builders	male	29.0	172.4	83.1	8.4	Fahey, et al
	male	27.6	178.8	88.1	8.3	Pipes
Wrestling	male	26.0	177.8	81.8	9.8	Fahey. et al
	male	27.0	176.0	75.7	10.7	Gayle, Flynn
	male	22.0	—	—	5.0	Parizkova
	male	23.0	—	79.3	14.3	Taylor, et al
	male	19.6	174.6	74.8	8.8	Sinning
	male	15-18	172.3	66.3	6.9	Katch, Michael
	male	20.6	174.8	67.3	4.0	Stine, et al

[1]Adapted from Wilmore, J.H. Training for Sport and Activity: The Physiological Basis of the Conditioning Process. 2nd ed. Boston: Allyn & Bacon, 1982. The complete references are provided in this source. To convert to inches and pounds, divide height in centimeters by 2.54, and multiply weight in kilograms by 2.205.
[2]professional athletes

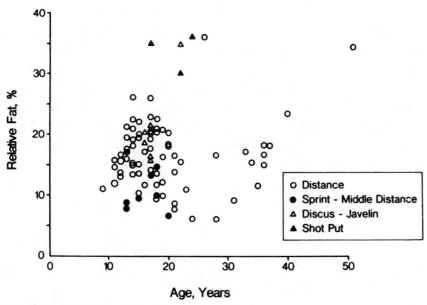

FIGURE 8. Relative body fat values for female track and field athletes.

SUMMARY

It is apparent that not only body weight, but more importantly, body composition, is a critical factor to the success of the athlete. Identifying the appropriate body composition for the athlete and then assigning a corresponding competitive weight for that athlete to attain and/or maintain, is now considered to be an essential part of the total management process. First, the coach, trainer, or team physician should select the most appropriate technique for estimating the athlete's body composition. Second, an acceptable range of values should be established, allowing for individual differences and for potential errors in the technique. Third, the athletes should be evaluated and provided with a suggested competitive weight, and a comprehensive dietary and exercise program which will allow the attainment of the suggested weight within a reasonable period of time, losing not more than 2 pounds per week. Finally, periodic re-evaluations should be scheduled to assure the coach and athlete, as well as the trainer and physician, that the suggested weights and body composition are being attained and maintained. This last point is particularly important when major changes in weight are observed. If the athlete undergoes a 20 pound weight gain or loss, it is imperative to know if the gain has been in lean tissue and the loss in body fat. To gain fat weight and lose lean weight is inconsistent with the stated objectives of the weight gain or weight loss program, i.e. to optimize body composition for that sport and to improve performance.

REFERENCES

1. Behnke, A.R. and J.H. Wilmore. **Evaluation and Regulation of Body Build and Composition.** Englewood Cliffs, NJ: Prentice-Hall, 1974.

2. Jackson, .A.S. and M.L. Pollock. Generalized equations for predicting body density in men. **Br. J. Nutr.** 40: 497-504, 1978.

3. Jackson, A.S., M.L. Pollock, and A. Ward. Generalized equations for predicting body density of women. **Med. Sci. Sports Exercise** 12:175-182, 1980.

4. Parizkova, J. Total body fat and skinfold thickness in children. **Metabolism** 10: 794-807, 1961.

5. Wilmore, J.H. **Training for Sport and Activity: The Physiological Basis of the Conditioning Process.** 2nd ed. Boston: Allyn & Bacon, 1982.

6. Wilmore, J.H. and W.L. Haskell. Body composition and endurance capacity of professional football players. **J. Appl. Physiol.** 33: 564-567, 1972.

7. Wilmore, J.H., R.B. Parr, W.L. Haskell, D.L. Costill, L.J. Milburn, and R.K. Kerlan. Athletic profile of professional football players. **Physician Sportsmed.** 4: 45-54, 1976.

Consequences of Rapid Weight Loss*

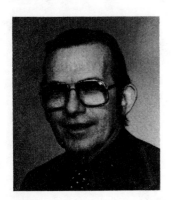

CHARLES M. TIPTON, PH.D.

Professor, Departments of Physical Education and Physiology and Biophysics, University of Iowa.
Editor-in-Chief of **Medicine and Science in Sports & Exercise.** Author of six books, numerous publications on mechanism of exercise adaptations. Past President, American College of Sports Medicine, and member, Orthopedic Research Society and American Physiological Society.

*Supported in part from funds provided by Iowa Medical Society and the Iowa High School Athletic Association

ABSTRACT

Wrestlers are unique as an athletic population because they deprive themselves of food and water to "make weight." Contrary to general impressions, scholastic or collegiate wrestlers are not fat prior to competiton. Of the dietary information they use, it originates from the "fellow wrestlers" and not from their parents, coaches or physicians. Most scholastic and collegiate wrestlers lose their weight in a brief period of time by water restriction combined with thermal and/or exercise dehydration. Relevant studies indicate this method of weight reduction will markedly decrease muscular endurance, tissue glycogen levels, muscle water content and impair the "normal" functioning of the cardiovascular and temperature regulation systems. Whether strength or aerobic capacity is altered is unclear; but, there is no evidence available which indicates a functional advantage will occur from this process. While there were no data to suggest that scholastic wrestlers became hypertensive from the making of weight, the urinary results clearly indicate they were dehydrated. Furthermore, we have speculated that the repeated periods of dehydration will result in acute and chronic conditions of renal ischemia. While long term research is needed to verify this postulate, parental, educational, scientific and medical groups must take prompt and bold action to change and modify these practices while educating coaches and participants on better and healthier ways to make weight.

There are few topics in Sports Medicine and Exercise Science that have as much interest, controversy and myths as nutrition and performance. Thus, it is appropriate that individuals with the different perspectives and backgrounds at this symposium re-examine this subject as we enter the decade of the 80s.

Of the myriad of athletic programs sponsored and sanctioned by educational associations and institutions, wrestling is the only sport that tacitly encourages weight loss before competition. Although educational and medical groups have repeatedly voiced their concerns during the past decades over the potential health hazards associated with this practice[3],[4],[5],[15], it continues. In fact, rules governing interscholastic wrestling state[28]:

> "The Rules Committee recommends the individual state high school associations develop and utilize an effective weight control program which will discourage severe weight reduction and/or wide variations in weight, because this may be harmful to the competitor. . ."

Weight reduction continues to be a problem primarily because of tradition, established weight classes, and an entrenched conviction that weight loss can occur without any decrement in performance. Our studies[16],[36][40],[44],[45] with Iowa scholastic and collegiate wrestlers (Figures 1-4) indicate that the majority of the body weight loss will occur in a relatively short period of time. For purposes of this presentation, we are discussing a body weight loss of 4-12 lbs. (1.8 - 5.4 kg) that will occur 2-48 hours before competition. This loss also represents a decrease from 2-12% in the body weight. Associated with these figures are findings that the youngest team members are also losing the highest percentages of their pre-competitive body weights[36]. The fact that the process will be repeated between 5-30 times a season should not be forgotten as we discuss the consequences[36],[37].

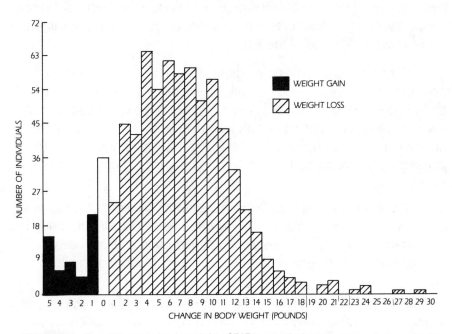

FIGURE 1: The changes in body weight of 747 Iowa scholastic wrestlers during a 17 day period. Printed with the permission of J. Iowa Med.Soc. 59:571-574, 1969.

Associated with these figures are findings that the youngest team members are also losing the highest percentages of their pre-competitive body weights[36]. The fact that the process will be repeated between 5-30 times a season should not be forgotten as we discuss the consequences[36],[37].

Previous speakers have effectively covered the importance of body

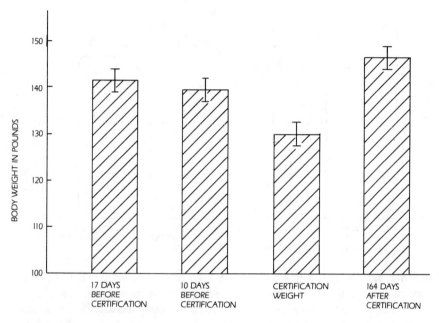

FIGURE 2. The time course of body weight changes in 126 Iowa scholastic wrestlers from six different high schools Means and standard errors are shown. Printed with the permission of the Journal of American Medical Society 214:1272, 1970.

compositional measurements in athletics. It is sufficient to reiterate that body weight is a unique composite of different fluids, minerals, electrolytes and tissues that can be conceptually classified into the components of lean body mass and fat (Table 1)[5,17,42,43]. Since numerous studies have indicated the oxidation of one pound (0.454 kg) of fat is approximately 3500 kcl and at an R of 1.00 the caloric equivalent of one liter of oxygen is essentially 5 kcl[6]; it is unlikely that the rapid weight loss preceding competition is due to fat oxidation. As demonstrated in the Minnesota starvation study[22], (Figure 5), food deprivation has a profound effect on performance. However, wrestlers utilize a variety of techniques

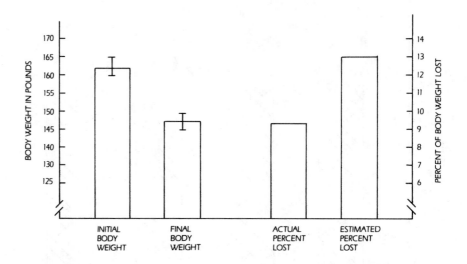

FIGURE 3. Body weight changes from 415 Iowa finalists during the 1972-73 season. The initial weight was the value on October 1 whereas the final weight was at the time of the tournament (late February). The estimated loss is the value which includes the two pound monthly weight allowance.

to "make weight" (Figure 4) and reduced caloric intake is not the only one selected prior to competition.

The primary means by which wrestlers lose weight is by dehydration. To enhance fluid loss, wrestlers exercise in hot environments by wearing warmup or rubber suits[37],[38]. However, it is important to realize that the spectrum of body compositional changes is altered when fluid restriction is combined with food deprivation[17], (Figure 6). Dehydration is a dilemma for the maintenance of fluid homeostasis because the body can not lose fluid and matintain both plasma volume and cellular hydration. Studies by a variety of investigators has demonstrated that changes in body fluids are influenced by (1) the rate of dehydration, (2) the presence of either a cool or

BODY COMPOSITION AND ATHLETIC PERFORMANCE

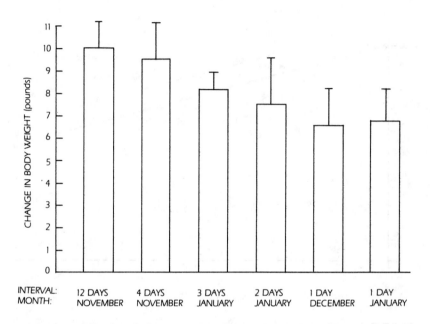

FIGURE 4. Body weight changes of collegiate varsity wrestlers during the season. Time interval refers to the duration prior to weigh in. Reprinted with permission of Medicine and Science in Sports 8:106, 1976.

a hot environment, (3) or whether the dehydration is due to a lack of water or to salt deprivation[1,2,18,24,27,31]. Contrary to earlier reports[23], Costill and associates have demonstrated that when the fluid loss exceeded four percent of the initial body weight, the loss was equally distributed among the intracellular and extracellular compartments[10,12].

The single most important effect of dehydration is a dramatic decrease in work capacity or endurance time[1,5,8,20,21,30,31,33]. This is true for either a cold or a warm environment[31]. Whether the acute changes in fluid loss will cause a decrease in muscular strength is debatable because no changes[33] as well as significant reductions[7,20] have been reported. Studies by Buskirk and assocaties[8] and Kataoka[20] have reported significant

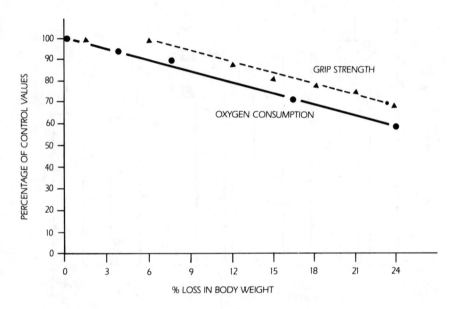

FIGURE 5. The influence of dietary restriction on muscle strength and aerobic capacity. Modified from the Minnesota starvation study data published by Taylor and Associates. J. Appl. Physiol. 10:421, 1957.

decreases in VO_2max although neither Saltin[33], Costill and Saltin[10], or Marrin et al.[25] could confirm this result in their investigations. The acute effects of making weight show declines in liver[19] and muscle glycogen levels[9,10,12,25]. In a preliminary report by Marrin and associates[25], muscle glycogen levels decreased by 48% in subjects who reduced their body weight by eight percent during a four day experimental period. The glycogen changes noted by Costill & Saltin[10,12] are of interest because they used thermal and exercise dehydration, methods frequently employed by wrestlers to lose weight.

Costill's et al. investigations[9,13] with various levels of dehydration (-2.2%, -4.1%, -5.8% BW) revealed that not only was muscle glycogen

BODY COMPOSITION AND ATHLETIC PERFORMANCE

TABLE 1. The Components of Lean Body Mass (%)

Muscle Tissue	47.6
Skeleton	15.9
Skin	13.5
Blood	8.6
G-I tract	3.6
Liver	2.7
Brain and Spinal Cord	2.3
Lungs	1.5
Heart	0.6
Essential fat	0.6
Kidney	0.5
Spleen	0.2
Pancreas	0.1
Miscellaneous and fat free adipose tissue	2.3
	100.0

Modified from Behnke, A.R., In Techniques for Measuring Body Composition. Edited by J. Brozek and A. Henschel, Washington, D.C. National Academy of Sciences, 1961, p. 121.

significantly decreased; but intracellular muscle water content as well. They noted a 1.2% decrease for each one percent decrease in body weight. Muscle sodium and chloride levels were unchanged while muscle potassium levels were increased. Using indirect methods, they calculated the resting muscle membrane potential and found no differences existed between the experimental conditions[9,10,12].

Adolph's earlier studies[1,31] have lead to the concept that fluid losses that are less than two percent of the initial body weight will have minimal effect on the functioning of the cardiovascular system. When losses exceed that value, notable changes are seen with sub-maximal work conditons which cause elevations in heart rate, decreases in stroke

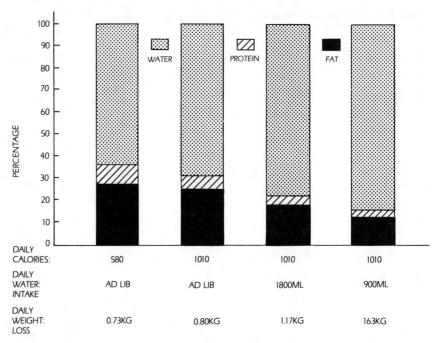

F. Grande, Techniques for Measuring Body Composition, 185, 1961

FIGURE 6. The influence of caloric restriction and water deprivation on body compositional changes. Redrawn from F. Grande in reference 17.

volume, and declines in cardiac output[34]. It is quite possible that myocardial contractility is decreased but further research is needed to verify this impression. There is little doubt that dehydration by exercise or by thermal methods will significantly reduce plasma volume, central blood volume and the distribution of blood to the active tissues[5,10,27,31,32,34].

Declines in plasma volumes ranging from six to 25 percent have been reported in subjects losing from three to eight percent of their initial body weight[9,10,31,34,41]. Body fluid losses not only influence cardiac output, they alter the temperature regulation system[27,31,32]. The volume of circulating blood is essential for the conductance of heat from the active tissues to the skin and the respiratory system where it will be dissipated[27],[31],[32]. Since many wrestlers exercise to lose weight, the evaporation of sweat becomes an important cooling mechanism. Unfortunately, sweating will be "shut down" when plasma volume decreases[27]. Therefore, exercising in a hot environment by dehydrated wrestlers who refuse to replenish their fluid losses is a potentially hazardous procedure because the reduction in the central circulatory volume coupled with decreased cooling will cause internal temperatures to increase. Dehydration must be considered as a serious problem to an athlete because for every one percent loss in body weight, the internal (core) body termpature will rise 0.17 to 0.28°C[42].

If strenuous exercise is performed in a hot environment and water loss is not replenished, a wrestler in the 150 pound weight class could lose between 3-5 pounds of fluid/hour (1.3 - 2.3 kg/hr). These conditions can lead to exhaustion, heat pyrexia, heat stroke and interference with the ability for temperature regulation[1],[31]. From the classical studies on the physiological effects of dehydration[1] it is possible to recognize signs of dehydration exhaustion (decreased work output, drowsiness, faintness, dyspnea, dry mouth and restlessness) that occur with progressive water loss[27],[31].

Fluids represent approximately 66% of the body weight of young male subjects. A 150 lb. wrestler has approximately 29 liters of intracellular fluid, 18 liters of extracellular fluids and 9 liters of interstitial fluids. The studies and calculations of Costill and Saltin[10] concerned fluid and electrolyte changes are relevant to this topic because they suggested 71% of the total weight loss by thermal or exercise dehydration originated from plasma and from intramuscular water. Costill also has reported that with a six percent loss in body weight by dehydration, eight percent of the total exchangeable sodium and chloride and one percent of the body stores for potassium and magnesium are lost[9].

Although the mechanisms are complex, it is well recognized that the

FIGURE 7. Urinary results from Iowa finalists prior to the weigh in and before the first match. Means and standard errors are shown. Controls were students from a local high school who did not participate in athletics. Original methods, data and results can be found in reference 45.

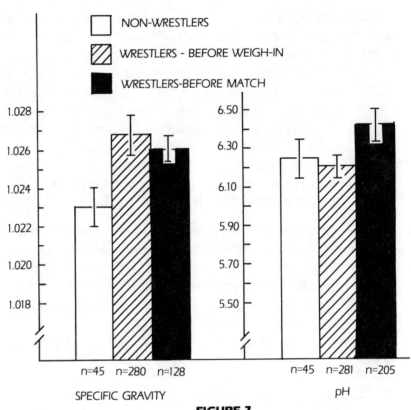

FIGURE 7.
A: Urinary specific gravity and pH results.

TABLE 2. Urinary Changes in Varsity Wrestlers Prior to Competition

Condition	Volume (ml/24h4)	Specific Gravity	pH	Osmolarity (mOsmol/l)	"Na" (MEg/24 hr)	"K" MEq/24 hr)	Creatinine (mg/24 hr)	LAP Activity G-R units/24 hr)
Day before Competition	816±188(7)	1.025±.002(8)	6.13±0.17(8)	865±75.0(8)	86.9±13.1(7)	59.1±17.4(7)	1359±267(7)	22.8±5.3(12)
Day of Competition	755±325(6)	1.029±0.002(7)	5.84±0.18(7)	959±46.9(7)	69.5±29.8(6)	50.3±8.2(6)	1629±409(5)	50.3±15.2(11)

Values are means and SE, the number of subjects is in parenthesis. Additional information can be obtained from reference 44.

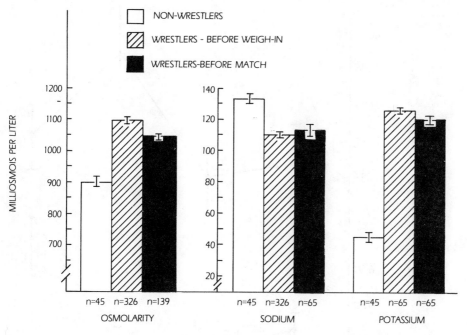

B. Urinary osomalarity, sodium and potassium levels.

FIGURE 7. Urinary results from Iowa finalists prior to the weigh in and before the first match. Means and standard errors are shown. Controls were students from a local high school who did not participate in athletics. Original methods, data and results can be found in reference 45.

kidneys play an important role in the regulation of body fluids and their electrolyte concentrations. Dehydration as well as strenuous exercise will cause decreases in renal blood flow, glomerular filtration rate, electrolyte concentrations, urine flow and levels of circulating hormones[5,9,29,31,35]. The urinary changes noted in Figures 7-9 and Tables 2 and 3 showed that both the scholastic and collegiate wrestlers were dehydrated at the weigh-in, prior to competition, during days of repeated competition and that three hours was an insufficient time for fluid and electrolyte restoration to

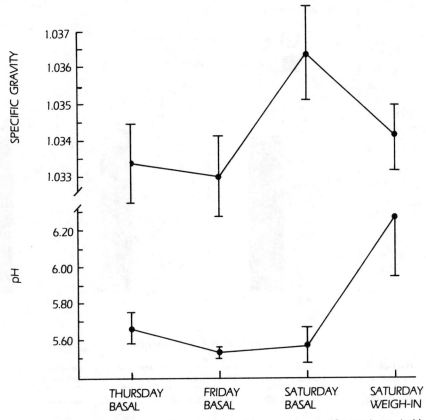

A. Urinary changes in varsity wrestlers with regard to specific gravity and pH.

FIGURE 8. Urinary changes in 24 hour samples collected from collegiate varsity wrestlers prior to competition. Means and standard errors listed. Printed with permission of Medicine and Science in Sports 8:105-108, 1976.

equilbrium conditions. This latter conclusion is also supported by other data[13],[41]. The changes in urinary leucine-amino-pepidase (LAP)[26] and the differential between urinary sodium and potassium concentrations during the various time periods represented in Figures 7-9 and Table 2,

BODY COMPOSITION AND ATHLETIC PERFORMANCE

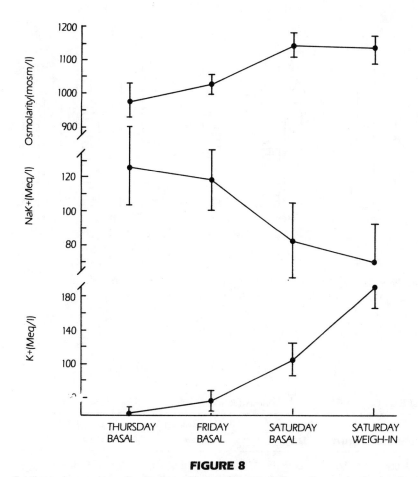

FIGURE 8. Urinary changes in 24 hour samples collected from collegiate varsity wrestlers prior to competition. Means and standard errors listed. Printed with permission of Medicine and Science in Sports 8:105-108, 1976.

FIGURE 8

B: Urinary changes in varsity wrestlers with regard to osmolarity, sodium and potassium levels.

have lead to the speculation that renal ischemia is frequently occurring during the acute stages of making weight[37],[44],[45]. Animal studies and investigations with isolated perfused kidneys have demonstrated that conditions of water deprivation, starvation and decreases in O_2 availability

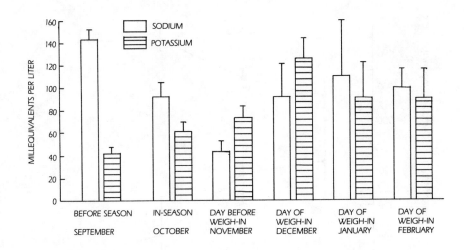

FIGURE 9. Urinary changes in sodium and potassium levels from collegiate varsity wrestlers prior to competition. The methods used and other findings can be found in reference 44.

TABLE 3. Urinary Changes in Finalists During a Three Day Period.

Parameter	Units	Initial Day	Second Day	Final Day
Osmolarity	nM/l	1069±135(136)	1051±133(111)	1124±154(98)
pH	-log H+	6.27±0.78(136)	5.97±0.79(111)	5.57±0.41(97)
Specific Gravity		1.028±0.005(108)	1.028±0.005(69)	1.027±0.006(68)
Na	Meq/L	128±68(135)	110±55(111)	96±44(98)
K	Meq/L	138±51(135)	111±48(111)	59±26(98)

Values are means and standard deviations; the number of animals is in parenthesis. All wrestlers were measured at the time of the official weigh-in, each had wrestled one or more matches by day two or three.

TABLE 4. Resting Blood Pressure Value of Wrestling Finalist Prior to Weigh-In

Parameter	Value	N
Systolic	115±1.0	101
Diastolic (Fourth Phase)	75±0.6	101
Diastolic (Fifth Phase)	61±0.8	98
Mean	93±0.7	101

Means and SE listed, wrestlers were measured in separate rooms under "quiet" conditions one hour before and after the official weight-in procedure.

TABLE 5. Minimal Caloric Requirements of Scholastic Wrestlers

Weight Class	N	Height In Inches	Age	Estimated Surface Area	Estimated Basal Calories Needed Per 24 Hours
98	30	62.6	15.0	1.42	1544
107	34	64.7	15.4	1.54	1674
115	50	65.7	15.5	1.60	1728
123	46	66.6	15.9	1.66	1781
130	54	67.5	15.8	1.70	1824
137	46	68.2	15.8	1.78	1910
145	46	68.1	15.9	1.82	1952
155	53	70.2	16.1	1.88	2017
165	39	70.2	16.3	1.94	2081
175	20	70.8	16.5	1.98	2100
185	16	70.5	16.5	2.08	2206

Results were from 434 Iowa high school wrestlers certified for competition.

will be associated with an increased release of potassium and elevated levels of LAP[14],[26],[44],[45]. While more research and direct measurements are needed, these results do raise the question as to whether repeated episodes of dehydration will cause anatomical and/or functional changes that could be manifested at a later date.

Because renal ischemia has been associated with the development of renal hypertension, resting blood pressures were obtained on selected finalists prior to and immediately after the weigh-in (Table 4). There were no findings that suggested that scholastic wrestlers were hypertensive as a group.

For our results and those of others, we have taken the position that the physiological and psychological consequences of acute weight loss in wrestlers are of sufficient importance to deserve prompt and immediate action by parental, educational and medical groups. Specifically, we feel wrestlers:

1. Must be educated and inculcated to replace fluids as they are lost and that they must compete in a hydrated state.

2. Must be educated that an adequate and balanced diet is essential for competition. Inherent in this statement is the understanding that the minimal caloric needs of an individual are dependent upon his age, surface area, and his daily energy expenditure (Table 5). Parents, coaches, and physicians should inititate changes so that the "other wrestlers" are not the primary source for nutritional information[38].

3. Must be certified for weight classes that are determined by the number of available participants. In Iowa,[40] we found that of approximately 9,000 individuals, forty percent were certified for the 119-138 classes. We also believe the time has arrived for these weight classes to have more competitors per class[40].

4. Must be assigned to weight classes by their body compositional

measurements. Our recommendation is to discourage certification of individuals who have less than five percent fat[37]. Although research has yet to prove that this is a safe lower limit or that such an approach would be practical to implement, the time has arrived for new approaches and directions to be taken in this area.

REFERENCES

1. Adolph, E.F. **Physiology of Man in the Desert.** New York: Interscience Pub., 1947.

2. Adolph, E.F. Tolerance to heat and dehydration in several species of mammals. **Am. J. Physiol.** 151:564-575, 1947.

3. AMA Committee on the Medical Aspects of Sports, Wrestling and Weight Control. **JAMA** 201:541-453, 1967.

4. AMA Statement: Weight Loss in Amateur Wrestling. Resolution 126, A-76. In House of Delegates, 1976, 2p.

5. American College of Sports Medicine position stand on weight loss in wrestlers. **Sports Medicine Bulletin** 11:1-2, 1976.

6. Astrand, P.O. and K. Rudahl. **Textbook of Work Physiology.** New York: McGraw Hill, 1977.

7. Bosco, J.S., R.L. Terjung and J.E. Greenleaf. Effects of progressive hypohydration on maximal isometric muscular strength. **J. Sports Med. Phys. Fit.** 8:81-86, 1968.

8. Buskirk, E.R., P.F. Iampietro and D.E. Bass. Work performance after dehydration: effects of physical conditioning and heat acclimatization. **J. Appl. Physiol.** 12:189-194, 1958.

9. Costill, D.L. Muscle water and electrolytes during acute and repeated bouts of dehydration. In: **International Symposium on Sportsmen's Nutrition.** Warsaw, 1975, 1-

10. Costill, D.L. and B. Saltin. Muscle glycogen and electrolytes following exercise and thermal dehydration. In: **Metabolic Adaptation to Prolonged Physical Exercise.** Edited by H. Howald and J.R. Poortmans. Basel: Berkhauser Verlag, 1975, pp. 352-360.

11. Costill, D.L. and K.E. Sparks. Rapid fluid replacement following thermal dehydration. **J. Appl. Physiol.** 34:299-303, 1973.

12. Costill, D.L., R. Cote and W. Fink. Muscle water and electrolytes following varied levels of dehydration in man. **J. Appl. Physiol.** 40:6-11, 1976.

13. Costill, D.L., R. Cote, E. Miller, T. Miller and S. Wynder. Water and electrolyte replacement during repeated days of work in the heat. **Aviat. Space Environ. Med.** 46:795-800,1975.

14. Deuvaert, R.E., G.M. Watkins, J.R. Dmochowski and N.P. Couch. Surface potassium ions activity of the ischemic kidney. **Surg. Gynecol. Obst.** 136:429-432, 1973.

15. Eriksen, F.G. Interscholastic wrestling and weight control: Current plans and their loopholes. In: **Proceedings of the Eighth National Conference on the Medical Aspects of Sports.** Chicago: AMA, 1967, pp.34-39.

16. Gisolfi, C.V. and C.M. Tipton. How to 'make weight': Rubberized suit or the First Law of Thermodynamics. **Scholastic Wrestling News** 10:6-8, 1974.

17. Grande, F. Nutrition and energy balance in body composition studies. In: **Techniques for Measuring Body Composition.** Edited by J. Brozek and A. Henschel. Washington, D.C.. National Acad. Sci. & Nat. Res. Council, 1961, pp.168-188.

18. Hopper, J., J.R. Elkington and A.W. Winkler. Plasma volume of dogs in dehydration with and without salt loss. **J. Clin. Invest.** 23:111-117, 1944.

19. Hultman, E. and L. Nilsson. Liver glycogen as glucose-supplying source during exercise. In: **Limiting Factors of Physical Performance.** Edited by J. Keul. Stuttgart: Georg Thieme, 1973, pp. 179-189.

20. Kataoka, Y. Studies on the effects of rapid weight reduction in sports with weight classification system. Report 1. Effects of weight reduction on cardio-respiratory function and muscular strength of wrestlers. **The Proceedings of the Department of Physical Education College of General Education Unviersity of Tokyo,** 7:29-40, 1972.

21. Kataoka, Y. Studies on the effects of rapid weight reduction in sports with weight classification system. Report 2. Effects of weight reduction of muscular endurance and power of wrestlers. **The Proceedings of the Department of Physical Education College of General Education. University of Tokyo,** 7:41-48, 1972.

22. Keys, A.L., J. Brozek, A. Henschel, O. Mickelsen and H.L. Taylor. **The Biology of Human Starvation,** Minneapolis: U. of Minn. Press, 1, 1950, pp. 718-748.

23. Kozlowski, S. and B. Saltin. Effect of sweat loss on body fluids. **J. Appl. Physiol.** 19:1119-1124, 1964.

24. MacFarland, W.V., R.J.H. Morris, B. Howard, J. McDonald and O.E. Budtz-Olsen. Water and electrolyte changes in tropical Merino sheep exposed to dehydration during summer. **Aust. J. Agr. Res.** 12:889-912, 1961.

25. Marrin, D.A., M.E. Houston, J.A. Thomson and H.J. Green. Physiological and metabolic effects of rapid weight reduction. **Med. Sci. Sports Exercise** 12:108, 1980.

26. Mason, E.E., F.A. Chernigoy, R.E. Caldwell and J.P. Burke. Clinical study of mild renal ischemia. **Surg. Gynecol. Obst.** 119-293-301, 1964.

27. Nadel, E.R. Temperature regulation. In: **Sports Medicine and Physiology.** Edited by R.H. Straus. Philadelphia: W.B. Saunders, 1979, pp. 130-146.

28. **The National Federation 1974-75 Wrestling Rule Book.** The National Federation Publications, Elgin, Illinois, p. 6.

29. Radigan, L.R. and S. Robinson. Effect of environmental heat stress and exercise on renal blood flow and filtration rate. **J. Appl. Physiol.** 2:185-191, 1949.

30. Ribisl, P.M. and W.G. Herbert. Effect of rapid weight reduction and subsequent rehydration upon the physical working capacity of wrestlers. **Res. Quart.** 41:536-541, 1970.

31. Robinson, S. The effect of dehydration on performance. In: **Football Injuries.** Washington: Nat. Acad. Sci., 1970, pp. 191-197.

32. Rowell, L.B. Human cardiovascular adjustment to exercise and thermal stress. **Physiol. Rev.** 54:75-159, 1974.

33. Saltin, B. Aerobic and anaerobic work capacity after dehydration. **J. Appl. Physiol.** 19:1114-1118, 1964.

34. Saltin, B. Circulatory response to submaximal and maximal exercise after thermal dehydration. **J. Appl. Physiol.** 19:1125-1132, 1964.

35. Smith, J.H., S. Robinson and M. Pearcy. Response to exercise, heat and dehydration. **J. Appl. Physiol.** 4:659-665, 1952.

36. Tcheng, T.K. and C.M. Tipton. Iowa wrestling study: anthrpometric measurements and the prediction of a 'minimal' body weight for high school wrestlers. **Med. Sci. Sports.** 5:1-10, 1973.

37. Tipton, C.M. Physiologic problems associated with the "making of weight." **Am. J. Sports Med.** 8:449-450, 1980.

38. Tipton, C.M. and T.K. Tcheng. Iowa wrestling study: Weight loss in

high school students. **JAMA** 2114:1269-1274, 1970.

39. Tipton, C.M., T.K. Tcheng and W.D. Paul. Evaluation of the Hall Method for determining minimum wrestling weights. **J. Iowa Med. Soc.** 59:571-574, 1969.

40. Tipton, C.M., T.K. Tcheng and E.J. Zambraski. Iowa wrestling study: Weight classification systems. **Med. Sci. Sports** 8:101-104, 1976.

41. Vaccaro, P., C.W. Zauner and J.R. Cade. Changes in body weight, hematocrit and plasma protein concentration due to dehydration and rehydration in wrestlers. **Med. Sci. Sports** 7:76, 1975.

42. Wilmore, J.H. **Athletic Training and Physical Fitness.** Boston: Allyn and Bacon, Inc. 1976, 118-139, 152-158, 200-215.

43. Wilmore, J.H. and A. Behnke. An anthropometric estimation of body density and lean body weight in young men. **J. Appl. Physiol.** 27:25-31, 1969.

44. Zambraski, E.J., D.T. Foster, P.M. Gross and C.M. Tipton. Iowa wrestling study: Weight loss and urinary profiles of collegiate wrestlers. **Med. Sci. Sports** 8:105-108, 1976.

45. Zambraski, E.J., C.M. Tipton, T.K. Tcheng, H.R. Jordan, A.C. Vailas and A.K. Callahan. Changes in the urinary profiles of wrestlers prior to and after competiton. **Med. Sci. Sports** 7:217-220, 1975.

ACKNOWLEDGMENT

These studies were accomplished with the able assistance of Drs. T.K. Tcheng and E.J. Zambraski.

Summary

Dr. Wilmore emphasized that body composition, rather than just body weight, is particularly important in assessing the appropriate body build for optimal athletic performance. Obviously, absolute body size is important for some events—we do not expect a football lineman to be the same size as a cross-country runner—but their body composition (relative percents of fat and lean tissue) could be similar.

The discussion brought out that a majority of well-conditioned men athletes have fat percentages above 9%-10%, with a "sort of average" in the 12% to 15% range. Women athletes tend to be 3% to 6% higher on the average. It also was suggested that a relative fat limit of about 6% to 8% was close to a lower limit for maintenance of adequate body reserves. Particular concern was expressed regarding the potential detrimental effect of very low body fat levels on the menstrual function of young female athletes. The mechanism by which low body fat alters menstrual function has not been established, nor have body composition criteria for optimal health and performance of young female endurance athletes.

The validity and accuracy of various techniques for assessing body composition were discussed, with the general consensus that hydrostatic weighing with direct measurement of residual lung volume was the best procedure available. The need for population specific formulas when estimating body composition from anthropometric measurements was stressed—formulas need to be sex, age and activity specific.

During the discussion, most of the participants agreed with Dr. Tipton that any large and rapid weight loss was potentially detrimental for the young athlete, since much of this loss is achieved by dehydration, which could have a negative influence on health as well as performance. In addition, some of this weight loss will be achieved by a reduction in lean body mass, which also would have a negative effect on muscular strength, power and endurance.

Unfortunately, no guidelines have been generally adopted by

athletic associations for maximal rapid weight loss permitted immediately prior to athletic competition, especially high school and college wrestling. The practice of "making weight" through dehydration and severe dieting is one of the major abuses still prevalent in organized athletics in the United States. Similar concern was expressed for young female dancers, figure skaters and gymnasts, who use starvation-type diets and dehydration to achieve "competition weight" or desired appearance.

SPECIAL PROBLEMS

Sports Anemia And Its Impact On Athletic Performance

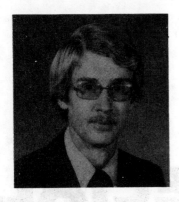

RUSSEL R. PATE, PH.D.

Director, Human Performance Laboratory, College of Health, University of South Carolina.
Associate Professor, Department of Physical Education. Fellow, American College of Sports Medicine and Research Consortium, American Alliance for Health, Physical Education, Recreation and Dance.

INTRODUCTION

Anemia is a condition characterized by a lower than normal concentration of hemoglobin in the blood. Since hemoglobin plays a central role in the blood's oxygen transport function, anemia can reduce oxygen delivery to body tissues and thereby impair the tissues' aerobic metabolic processes. Indeed, severe anemia is often associated with symptons such as chronic fatigue and listlessness.

In recent years several researchers and clinicians have reported observation of anemia in some athletes, particularly those involved in endurance activities such as distance running[12], [19], [36]. Thus the term "sports anemia" has entered the sports medicine lexicon. Since endurance performance is dependent largely on aerobic energy yielding processes, it seems clear that anemia could impair athletic performance in activities which require high levels of cardiorespiratory endurance. As such, sports anemia has been a focus of concern for athletes, coaches and sports medicine specialists.

This paper is intended to provide a critical analysis of currently available information on sports anemia. Specifically, the following questions will be addressed: what is sports anemia and how might it affect the endurance athlete?; how prevalent is sports anemia?; what are the possible causes of anemia in athletes?; how can sports anemia be prevented or treated?; how does hemoglobin concentration relate to endurance athletic performance?; and, how should the practitioner approach the sports anemia issue?

ENDURANCE EXERCISE, OXYGEN TRANSPORTATION AND ANEMIA

In recent years a massive number of scientific investigations have been directed toward identification of the factors which affect the performance of endurance exercise in man. These studies have led to the conclusion that an individual's endurance performance reflects a multiplicity of physiological, biochemical, biomechanical and psychological variables. One physiological variable which is known to correlate strongly with endurance performance is maximal aerobic power (VO_2max).

VO_2max, the maximum rate of oxygen utilization, determines the athlete's peak rate of aerobic energy expenditure. Since the anaerobic energy systems have very limited capacities, the aerobic metabolic processes must provide most of the energy for sustained moderate-to-high intensity exercise. Thus, the rates at which an athlete can expend energy and perform work for prolonged periods are determined largely by the VO_2max. In tangible terms, VO_2max is the best single predictor of the fastest pace at which an athlete can run, swim or cycle for extended periods of time.

During vigorous exercise, oxygen is consumed primarily in the active skeletal muscle fibers. These fibers are endowed with the metabolic machinery needed to release energy from foodstuffs via oxidation. Since the muscle fibers' capacity for oxygen storage is quite small, the cardiorespiratory system must continually replenish the muscles' supply of oxygen. Athough the factors which limit VO_2max have long been debated, the majority of exercise physiologists have viewed the cardiorespiratory system's maximal rate of oxygen delivery to the muscles as the principle determinant of VO_2max. Oxygen delivery to a muscle is a function of: (1) rate of blood flow through the muscle, and (2) the oxygen carrying capacity of the blood. The latter variable is determined primarily by the blood's hemoglobin concentration. Thus, a low hemoglobin concentration could reduce the maximal rate of oxygen delivery to tissues and, thereby, decrease VO_2max and impair endurance performance.

DEFINITIONS OF SPORTS ANEMIA

As indicated in Table 1, the normal range for hemoglobin concentration is lower for females than males and is quite wide for both sexes. Traditionally, the clinically accepted criterion for anemia is a hemoglobin concentration below the normal range, i.e., below 12 g% in females or below 14 g% in males[5]. Thus, one definition of "sports anemia" is the observation of clinical anemia in an athlete or physically very active individual.

However, such a definition of sports anemia may not be entirely satisfactory. In the athletic situation emphasis is placed on maximizing performance. Since "normal" values for physiological variables may not be optimal in terms of athletic performance, we must consider the possibility that athletes should manifest hemoglobin concentrations well above the 12 or 14 g% which are considered acceptable for normal populations of females and males, respectively.

Designation of an optimal hemoglobin concentration for athletes requires consideration of the relationship between hematocrit and blood viscosity. Hematocrit, the percentage of the blood which is red blood cells, is highly correlated with hemoglobin concentration. Viscosity is a major determinant of the rate at which blood will flow through the vascular system. As shown in Figure 1, it is known that blood viscosity increases curvilinearly with increases in hematocrit. Exceptionally high hematocrits, such as observed in polycythemia, can result in reduced oxygen delivery to peripheral tissues because the blood's high oxygen carrying capacity is more than offset by a reduced rate of blood flow. Thus, we cannot simply conclude that, for hemoglobin concentration, higher is always better. In fact, cardiovascular physiologists have tended to agree that the optimal hematocrit falls near the upper end of the normal range, i.e., near 45%[27], [31],. A hematocrit of 45% corresponds to a hemoglobin concentration of approximately 16 g%.

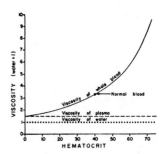

FIGURE 1. Relationship Between Hematocrit and Blood Viscosity.

In recent years this generalization regarding the optimal hemoglobin concentration has been challenged by two lines of research. First, studies on experimental enhancement of hemoglobin concentration by blood removal and subsequent reinfusion ("blood doping") have indicated that such treatments are associated with increases in maximal aerobic power and endurance performance[13], [15]. Second, recent investigations of the relationship between hematocrit and blood viscosity indicate that the optimal hemtocrit for oxygen delivery during exercise may be higher than previously supposed, perhaps as high as 50-60%[16]. These observations suggest that the optimal hemoglobin concentration for athletes may be at the upper end of the normal range. Thus, sports anemia could be defined as any hemoglobin concentration below that which is optimal for oxygen delivery. By this definition, any hemoglobin concentration below 15-16 g% could be interpreted as too low for the endurance athlete.

PREVALENCE OF SPORTS ANEMIA

Studies of the prevalence of sports anemia have utilized both epidemiological and experimental research designs. The epidemiological studies have been performed by assessing hematological variables in athletic populations. Tables 2 and 3 provide summaries of the epidemiological surveys of hemoglobin concentration in male and female athletes of various sport specialties and levels of competitive competency.

The data presented in Table 2 suggests that "low normal" hemoglobin concentration values are typical of male athletes, particularly those engaged in endurance sports. Anemia of the clinically significant nature (hemoglobin concentration less than 14 g%) is apparently quite rare. In women, identification of a pattern is more difficult since fewer data are available. The data presented in Table 3 suggest that mean hemoglobin concentrations for women athletes approximate those for the non-athletic population of adult women.

Several authors have employed an experimental model in observing the effects of heavy training on hematological variables. Yoshimura has suggested that a transient anemia may occur with the onset of chronic endurance training[36], however, this hypothesis does not appear to be extensively documented. Davis and Brewer did observe a transient anemia during the first few weeks of endurance training in dogs[9]. In humans, Lindemann[23] and Oscai[25] have reported observations of reduced hemoglobin concentrations with training and Dressendorfer[12] observed substantial decreases in hemoglobin concentration in runners participating in a 20 day road race. In contrast, Kilbom[22] found no change in hemoglobin concentration in adult women exposed to endurance training and Glass[18] reported no change in hemoglobin in cyclists who underwent a marked increase in training load. At present, only the following tentative conclusion can be drawn: heavy training may cause a transient anemia during the initial weeks of exercise; in the longer term, hemoglobin concentration in athletes seems to maintain a steady state in the mid to lower levels of the normal range.

TABLE 1. Hemoglobin Concentration in Adult Males and Females

	Normal Range for Hemoglobin Concentration	Clinical Criteria for Anemia
Males	14-18 g%	<14 g%
Females	12-16 g%	<12 g%

TABLE 2. Hematological Status of Male Athletes

Author	Group	N	Hemoglobin (G%)
Clement (4)	Canadian Olympians	123	14.7
	Canadian Norm		15.5±1.8
Dewijn (10)	Dutch Olympians	136	15.5±1.0
	Officials	36	15.8±1.1
Stewart (30)	Australian Olympians (E)	23	15.8±0.8
	Australian Olympians (NE)	13	16.9±0.8
Brotherhood (2)	Distance Runners	39	14.6±0.7
	Controls	12	15.1±1.0
	Elite Runners	20	15.5±0.9
Martin (24)	Good Runners	8	15.6±0.7
	Controls	95	15.8±1.1
Ehn (14)	Distance Runners	8	14.9±0.4
Hunding (21)	Runners, Joggers	80	14.5±1.0

TABLE 3. Hematological Status of Female Athletes

Author	Group	N	Hemoglobin (G%)
Clement (4)	Canadian Olympians	64	12.9
	Canadian Norm		13.6±1.6
Dewijn (10)	Dutch Olympians	43	14.4±0.8
Hunding (21)	Runners, Joggers	33	13.1±1.6
Pate (26)	College Athletes	46	14.6±0.9
Stewart (30)	Australian Olympians	6	15.5±0.3

POSSIBLE CAUSES OF SPORTS ANEMIA

Reports of suboptimal hemoglobin levels in athletes have generated much speculation regarding the possible causes of sports anemia. Since clinical anemia in the general population is often associated with nutritional deficiencies, several authors have suggested that sports anemia could be a result of inadequate dietary practices in athletes. Particular attention has been focused on possible problems associated with iron metabolism.

Substantial evidence indicates that certain athletic groups maintain lower than normal body iron stores. For example, Dufaux[13], Ehn[14] and Hunding[21] have reported observation of low iron stores in male runners. Likewise, several authors have reported low iron stores in selected groups of female athletes[19, 21, 22]. Low iron storage is generally considered to be a risk factor for anemia. Thus, the incidence of low iron stores in certain athletes is reasonably well documented. Regrettably, the causes of low iron storage in athletes are not well understood.

Low iron storage, which increases risk of anemia, could be due to: (1) inadequate dietary iron, (2) low absorption of iron from the digestive tract, and/or (3) high rates of iron loss. While it certainly is possible that some individual athletes do not receive adequate dietary iron, surveys of the dietary practices of athletes generally have shown athletes to have adquate iron intakes. For example, Steel[29] and Stewart[30] studied the nutritional practices of Australian 1968 Olympic athletes and found that iron intakes averaged over twice the recommended daily allowance. Further, it was reported that those athletes who manifested "suboptimal" hemoglobin levels were **not** characterized by low iron intakes. The finding that athletes obtain adequate dietary iron might well be expected since total caloric intake tends to be high in athletes.

Available evidence provides some support for the contention that some athletes experience low rates of iron absorption and high rates of iron loss. Ehn[14] found low rates of iron absorption and high rates of iron elimination in eight distance runners studied over two years. Vellar[33] has shown that iron losses through sweat can be substantial. In addition, it is well known that menstruating females experience a significant iron loss with each menstrual period. Several authors have suggested that athletes may experience high levels of intravascular hemolysis, i.e., rupture of red blood cells[21, 35, 36]. This may be a transient condition resulting from the breakdown of fragile red cells at the onset of heavy training[23, 36] or may be a chronic condition reflecting a continual damaging of red cells[7, 21]. Davidson has hypothesized that runners and joggers may inflict trauma on red cells circulating through the capillaries in the feet[7]. Mechanical destruction of red blood cells may be manifested as hemoglobinuria, the presence of free hemoglobin in the urine. This condition has been reported in some athletes, but its incidence does not appear to be high[7, 12].

One factor which probably contributes to the low hemoglobin concentration observed in many athletes is expansion of the plasma volume. It is well documented that endurance athletes manifest a relatively large total blood volume[2, 11] and that endurance training is accompanied by increases in plasma volume and total hemoglobin[20, 25]. However, decreases in hemoglobin concentration could result from an elevated plasma volume which is not matched by a proportional elevation of the red cell mass or total hemoglobin. This response was reported by Oscai[25] who exposed adult male subjects to sixteen weeks of running training. A similar observation was made by Brotherhood[2] who compared endurance runners with controls. Hemoglobin concentration was somewhat lower in the runners despite their manifestation of a total hemoglobin which was 20% greater than the controls. Thus, it seems likely that, in some athletes, training may result in a greater increase in plasma volume than total hemoglobin.

While many possible causes of sports anemia have been suggested, few have been studied in depth in athletic populations. Consequently, only a tentative conclusion can be drawn regarding the etiology of sports anemia. At present it appears that the "low normal" hemoglobin concentration which is characteristic of certain athletic groups is a result of elevated plasma volume perhaps complicated by increased rates of iron loss and red blood cell turnover. In some individual athletes these conditions may be complicated by low intake of dietary iron.

TREATMENT AND PREVENTION OF SPORTS ANEMIA

For a sports medicine practitioner the most important issues regarding sports anemia concern its treatment and/or prevention. The traditional approach to treatment of existing clinical-grade anemia has involved dietary iron therapy. Although no controlled studies of iron therapy in truly anemic athletes appear in the literature, enhancement of dietary iron would seem to be a reasonable first approach to treatment of true anemia in athletes. Gardner, et al.[17] have shown that iron therapy results in increased hemoglobin concentration and increased maximal aerobic power in anemic patients. Administration of iron could be expected to alleviate anemia in cases in which the condition has arisen due to low dietary iron or increased iron loss. However, treatment modalities other than iron therapy should be considered by the sports medicine specialist. In some cases, increased protein consumption[36] and modificiation of training programs may prove helpful.

Relatively little scientific investigation has been directed toward identification of methods for prevention of anemia in athletes. Pate, et al[26] and Cooter and Mowbray[6] studied the affects of season-long iron supplementation on hematological variables in female athletes. Both studies concluded that iron supplementation had no significant impact on the hematological status of the subjects, all of whom had normal hemoglobin levels prior to initiation of iron supplementation. Somewhat similar studies on iron supplementation have been reported by Weswig[34] and Bottiger[1] and in both cases the authors reported no significant effect on hemoglobin concentration. Based on these findings it seems inappropriate to recommend that all athletes ingest dietary iron supplements for prophylactic reasons. Yoshimura[36] has reported that protein supplementation can prevent anemia in athletes who are beginning heavy training, however, this conclusion was based on the results of a single study. Clearly, further study of the effects of dietary supplements on prevention of sports anemia is required.

IMPACT OF SPORTS ANEMIA ON ATHLETIC PERFORMANCE

There is little doubt that clinical-grade anemia is associated with impairment of endurance exercise performance. For example, Davies et al[8] observed low VO_2max values in moderately and severely anemic subjects. Sproule[28] found that the cardiorespiratory responses to exercise in anemia patients were approximately normal at low work loads but were adversely affected at high exercise intensities.

Unfortunately, the relationship between endurance performance and hemoglobin concentration is much less clear when only hemoglobin values in the normal range are considered. In a major study of hemoglobin concentration and maximal aerobic power, Vellar[32] found no significant relationship between hematological variables (within the normal range) and VO_2max expressed relative to body weight ($ml.kg^{-1}.min^{-1}$). It may be that, in such studies, the importance of hemoglobin concentration is obscured by the statistical weight of the many other variables which impact on VO_2max. This is suggested by the aforementioned studies which have used blood reinfusion to increase hemoglobin levels while endeavoring to hold other variables constant[3, 15]. Nonetheless, one must conclude that the functional significance of a "sub-optimal" or "low normal" hemoglobin concentration is, at present, unclear. This issue should be a focus of future research.

CONCLUSIONS

The information presented in the foregoing sections provides a basis for several conclusions regarding sports anemia:

1. The incidence of clinical-grade anemia in athletes is quite low and does not exceed that in the non-athletic population. However, a substantial percentage of athletes, particularly in endurance sports, manifest hemoglobin concentrations which might be classified as "sub-optimal".

2. A transient anemia may occur at the onset of heavy training. The mechanism underlying this phenomenon is not fully understood.

3. Many athletes, particularly those in endurance sports, manifest low iron stores and thus are at increased risk of developing anemia.

4. In certain athletes low dietary iron and/or protein intake, high levels of intravascular hemolysis and menstrual blood loss may increase risk of anemia.

5. Iron supplementation is usually an effective treatment for clinical-grade anemia. This and other treatment modalities such as training modifications should be considered when treating the anemic athlete. However, regular dietary iron supplementation does not appear warranted for purposes of preventing anemia in those athletes who are not at risk for its development.

6. Clinical-grade anemia is clearly associated with impaired endurance performance; however, the effects of "low normal" hemoglobin concentrations on endurance performance are less well understood.

In conclusion, it is apparent that the athletic population includes a small percentage of clinically anemic individuals and a larger percentage of persons who are at increased risk of its development. Future research should be directed toward development of improved methods for identifying athletes who are at significant risk of developing anemia. Also, more research is required to determine the significance, in athletes, of a so-called sub-optimal hemoglobin concentration.

REFERENCES

1. Bottiger, L.E., A. Nyberg, I. Astrand, et al. Jarntillforsel till friska studenter med hog fysisk aktivitet. **Nordisk Medin** 85:396, 1971.

2. Brotherhood, J., B. Brozovic and L.G.C. Pugh. Haematological status of middle-and long-distance runners. **Clin. Sci. Mol. Med.** 48:139, 1975.

3. Buick, F.J., N. Gledhill, A.B. Froese, L. Spriet and E.C. Meyers. Effect of induced erythrocythemia on aerobic work capacity. **J. Appl. Physiol.: Respirat. Environ. Exercise Physiol.** 48 (4): 636-642.

4. Clement, D.B., R.C. Asmundson and C.W. Medhurst. Hemoglobin values: comparative survey of the 1976 Canadian Olympic team. **Can. Med. Assoc. J.** 117: 614, 1977.

5. Committee on Iron Deficiency. Iron Deficiency in the United States. **JAMA** 203 (6): 119, 1968.

6. Cooter, G.R. and K.W. Mowbray. Effects of iron supplementation and activity on serum iron depletion and hemoglobin levels in female athletes. **Res Quart Am All Health Phys Ed Rec** 49:114, 1978.

7. Davidson, R.J.L. March or exertional haemoglobinuria. **Sem. Hemat.** 6:150, 1969.

8. Davies, C.T.M., A.C. Chukweumeka and J.P.M. Van Haaren. Iron-deficiency anaemia: its effect on maximum aerobic power and responses to exercise in African males aged 17-40 years. **Clin. Sci.** 44: 555, 1973.

9. Davis, J.E. and N. Brewer. Effect of physical training on blood volume, hemoglobin, alkali reserve and osmotic resistance of erythrocytes. **Am. J. Physiol.** 13: 586, 1935.

10. deWijn, J.R., J.L. deJongste, W. Mosterd, et al. Haemoglobin, packed cell volume, serum iron and iron binding capacity of selected athletes during training. **J. Sports Med. Phys. Fitness** 11:42, 1971.

11. Dill, D.B., K. Braithwaite, W.C. Adams, et al. Blood volume of middle-distance runners; effect of 2,300-m altitude and comparison witn non-athletes. **Med. Sci. Sports** 6:1, 1974.

12. Dressendorfer, R.H., C.E. Wade and E.A. Amsterdam. Development of a pseudoanemia in marathon runners during a 20-day road race. **JAMA** 246 (11): 1215, 1981.

13. Dufaux, B., A. Hoederath, I. Streitberger, et al. Serum ferritin, trans-ferrin haptoglobin and iron in middle-and long-distance runners, elite rowers and professional racing cyclists. **Int. J. Sports Medicine** 2: 43, 1981.

14. Ehn, L., B. Carlmark and S. Hoglund. Iron status in athletes involved in intense physical activity. **Med. Sci. Sports Exercise** 12: 61, 1980.

15. Ekblom, B., A.N. Goldbarg and B Gullbring. Response to exercise after blood loss and refinfusion. **J. Appl. Physiol.** 33: 175, 1972.

16. Gaehtgens, P., F. Kreutz and K.H. Albrecht. Optimal hematocrit for canine skeletal muscle during rhythmic isotonic exercise. **Eur. J. Appl. Physiol.** 4: 27, 1979.

17. Gardner, G.W., V.R. Edgerton, R.J. Barnard, et al. Cardiorespiratory, hematological and physical performance responses of anemic subjects to iron therapy. **Am. J. Clin. Nutr.** 28: 982, 1975.

18. Glass, H.I., R.H.T. Edwards, A.C. DeGarreta, et al. [11]CO red cell labeling for blood volume and total hemoglobin in athletes: effect of training. **J. Appl. Physiol.** 26: 131, 1969.

19. Haynes, E.M. Iron deficiency and the active woman. In: **DGWS Research Reports, Women in Sports,** vol. 2. Washington: AAHPER Press, 1973.

20. Holmgren, A., F. Mossfeldt, T. Sjostrand, et al. Effect of training on work capacity, total hemoglobin, blood volume, heart volume and pulse rate in recumbent and upright positions. **Acta Physiol. Scand.** 19: 146, 1949.

21. Hunding, A., R. Jordal and P.E. Paulev. Runner's anemia and iron deficiency. **Acta Med. Scand.** 209: 315, 1981.

22. Kilbom, A. Physical training with submaximal intensities in women. I. reaction to exercise and orthostasis. **Scand. J. Clin. Lab. Invest.** 28: 141, 1971.

23. Lindemann, R. Low hematocrits during basic training: athlete's anemia: **New Eng. J. Med.** 299: 1191, 1978.

24. Martin, R.P., W.L. Haskell and P.D. Wood. Blood chemistry and lipid profiles of elite distance runners. **Annals N.Y. Acad. Sci.** 301: 346, 1977.

25. Oscai, L.B., B.T. Williams and B.A. Hertig. Effect of exercise on blood volume. **J. Appl. Physiol.** 24: 622, 1968.

26. Pate, R.R., M. Maguire and J.Van Wuk. Dietary iron supplementation in women athletes. 7(9): **Physician and Sportsmedicine** 81, 1979.

27. Richardson, T.Q. and A.C. Guyton. Effects of polycythemia and anemia on cardiac output and other circulatory factors. **Am. J. Physiol.** 197: 1167, 1959.

28. Sproule, B.J., J.H. Mitchell and W.F. Miller. Cardiopulmonary physiological responses to heavy exercise in patients with anemia. **J. Clinc. Invest.** 39: 378, 1960.

29. Steel, J.E. A nutritional study of Australian olympic athletes. **Med. J. Austral.** 2(3): 119, 1970.

30. Stewart, G.A., J.E. Steel, A.H. Toyne, et al. Observations on the haematology and the iron and protein intake of Australian olympic athletes. **Med. J. Austral.** 2: 1339, 1972.

31. Stone, H.O., H.K. Thompson and K. Schmidt-Neilsen. Influence of erythrocytes on blood viscosity. **Am. J. Physiol.** 214: 913, 1968.

32. Vellar, O.D. and L. Hermansen. Physical performance and hematological parameters. **Acta Med. Scand. Suppl.** 522: 1, 1971.

33. Valler, O.D. Studies on sweat losses of nutrients. I. Iron content of whole body sweat and its association with other sweat constitutents, serum iron levels, hematological indices, body surface area, and sweat rate. **Scand. J. Clin. Lab. Invest.** 21: 157, 1968.

34. Weswig, P.H. and W. Winkler. Iron supplementation and hematological data of competitive swimmers. **J. Sports Med. Phys. Fitness** 14: 112, 1974.

35. Williamson, M.R. Anemia in runners and other athletes. **Physician and Sportsmedicine** 9(8): 73, 1981.

36. Yoshimura, H. Anemia during physical training (sports anemia). **Nutr. Rev.** 28: 251, 1970.

The Diabetic Patient and Athletic Performance

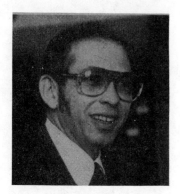

ARTHUR S. LEON, M.S., M.D.

Professor, Laboratory of Physiological Hygiene, Division of Health and Human Behavior, School of Public Health, University of Minnesota.
Director of Laboratories and Applied Research, Nutrition Trial Center.
Attending physician and consultant, Department of Medicine, Division of Clinical Pharmacology and Cardiology, University of Minnesota Medical School. Consultant to HEW and National Institute of Health.

PREVALENCE AND INCIDENCE

Diabetes is one of the major health problems facing our nation. It is a common disorder whose prevalence appears to be steadily increasing. About 5 million Americans have known diabetes, and it is estimated that an additional 4 to 5 million probably have undiagnosed diabetes.[1, 2] The prevalence and incidence rate increases with age. The rates are higher in non-whites than in the white population with the prevalence reaching a peak level of 10.5% among non-whites age 65 and over. Diabetes is also 50% more frequently in females than in males.

The disease ranks as the sixth leading cause of mortality in the United States. It is the direct underlying cause of about 40,000 deaths annually and this rate is steadily increasing. These data actually seriously underestimate the contribution of diabetes to mortality since many persons with diabetes die as a result of vascular complications related to their diabetes (mainly heart attacks or strokes). In addition to vascular complications, diabetes is an important contributor to visual impairment, blindness, and kidney disease in the United States.

SPECIAL PROBLEMS

DEFINITIONS AND DESCRIPTION[2-4]

Diabetes mellitus is one of the oldest diseases known to man. It was described in India in 400 BC, and in the fourth century BC in the Egyptian Ebers Papyrus. Ancient Greek physicians first coined the term "diabetes" meaning to run through a siphon; the Latin word "mellitus", meaning honey was added much later. For centuries after the discovery of "honey urine", physicians diagnosed the disease by tasting the patient's urine for sweetness, a forerunner of the modern laboratory analysis for sugar (glucose) in the urine.

In actuality diabetes mellitus is a group of metabolic disorders having in common actual or relative insufficiency of insulin. The best known actions of insulin are its ability to promote the transport of glucose across the cell membrane and its subsequent oxidation. Thus, insulin insufficiency results in an inability to utilize glucose as a fuel. This leads to elevated levels in the blood (hyperglycemia), the clinical hallmark of this disease. When the level of blood glucose circulating through the kidney exceeds 160 to 180 mg/dl, it usually spills over into the urine (glycosuria). This is accompanied by increased frequency of urination and volume of urine excreted (polyuria). The associated loss of large amounts of body water increases sensation of thirst and water intake (polydipsia), however, dehydration may still result.

In addition to its effect on glucose uptake and utilization as a fuel, other metabolic actions of insulin include storage of glucose as glycogen in muscle and liver; fat (triglyceride) synthesis in adipose cells, and inhibition of its breakdown (antilipolytic effect); and protein synthesis and storage (anabolic effect). Insulin insufficiency thus leads to a host of metabolic derangements. These are reflected in development of the common symptons of fatigue, weakness, weight loss, hunger, and overeating (polyphagia).

Increased lipolysis of triglycerides in adipose tissues associated with insulin insufficiency raises the concentration of free fatty acids in the blood and their use for fuel. The liver has a limited capacity to utilize acetylcoenzyme A generated from metabolism of FFA. Increased formation of the so-called ketone bodies results. These ketone bodies accumulate in the blood, spill over into the urine, and cause acidosis and dehydration and can lead to coma (ketoacidosis). Before the discovery of insulin, patients with severe ketoacidosis often did not survive. Now insulin replacement therapy helps correct the metabolic deficiency state, control the symptoms and signs of diabetes and prevents ketoacidosis.

TYPES OF DIABETES

Evidence that diabetes is a heterogeneous syndrome is derived from a variety of sources[3]. These include clinical and laboratory evidence that diabetes may result from a wide variety of mechanisms including other endocrine diseases and genetic disorders, heterogeneity of animal models, and differences in patterns of inheritance.

There are a number of systems for classification of individual types of diabetes mellitus.[3, 5] One way is by the stage of the disease:

1. **Potential Diabetes (Prediabetes).** This term describes situations in which future development of diabetes is anticipated because of a strong family history.

2. **Subclinical Diabetes.** This is defined as an abnormality in glucose tolerance in response to an oral or intravenous glucose challenge, but no clinical evidence of diabetes. Other terms often included under this heading are "asymptomatic", and "chemical" diabetes.

3. **Manfiest Diabetes or Clinical Diabetes.** These patients have typical symptoms and signs of diabetes.

4. **Brittle (labile) Diabetes.** These patients show wide swings between hyperglycemia and ketoacidosis on the one side and hypoglycema on

the other despite attempts to avoid them.

5. **Insulin-resistance Diabetes.** This group include diabetics who react to administration of insulin by high production of antibodies creating the need for excessively high doses of insulin for control.

A commonly used classification is that of the WHO Expert Committee. In the WHO classification, diabetes is divided into two major clinical types based primarily on age of onset: juvenile or growth-onset and maturity or adult-onset. Another commonly used classification is based on whether insulin therapy is required: Type I, insulin-dependent diabetes and Type II, non-insulin dependent diabetes. More elaborate classifications have been proposed taking etiological factors into consideration, but are still controversial and have not been universally accepted.

DIABETOGENIC FACTORS

Influence of Heredity. The inherited predispostion of diabetes has been established and appears to be more important in the juvenile type.[2-4] Indentical twins show a fourfold higher concordance for diabetes than non-identical twins. If both parents are diabetic the children have a 30% chance of eventually developing diabetes. Twelve percent of newly diagnosed diabetics have close relatives with diabetes as compared to 2% of non-diabetics. The relative frequency of certain blood groups and histocompatibility antigens (HLA) in juvenile diabetics, and genetically-linked diabetes in animals confirms genetic factors.[6] The present evidence suggests a multifactoral mode of inheritance.

Influence of Viruses and Autoimmune Mechanisms. In animal experiments it has been possible to induce diabetes by infection with certain viruses which destroy pancreatic islet cells.[3] In humans there is suggestive evidence that mumps and coxsackie B viruses can induce diabetes in a similar manner, however, this remains an open question.

A possibility also exists that viral damaged or destroyed islet cells may act as antigens. Antibodies may then be produced in susceptible individuals which destroy remaining beta cells.

Role of Obesity. Epidemiologic studies have shown that obesity is a major risk factor for development of maturity-onset diabetes. Incidence rates in the very obese are more than 20 times greater than in the non-obese.[1,2] About 80% of maturity-onset diabetics are obese. In contrast, the incidence rates are exceedingly low in lean individuals. Supporting evidence of the role of obesity in diabetes is the demonstration that weight gain and overweight may result in decreased activity of insulin (cellular resistance) due to loss of insulin receptors in distended adipose cells.[7,8] This can be reversed by loss of weight and body fat.

Role of Physical Inactivity. Epidemiologic studies have revealed that sedentary lifestyle is a very important risk factor for development of diabetes.[2] Most likely this is at least partially related to associated obesity. However, experimental evidence suggests an additional direct relationship. Inactivity as provided by bed rest within a few days leads to glucose intolerance and over-secretion of insulin apparently due to development of cellular resistance to insulin.[9] In addition, recent in vitro studies have revealed decreased numbers of insulin receptors in physically inactive as compared to active people, both diabetics and non-diabetics.[10–12]

Effect of Diet. A commonly held misconception is that diabetes results from excess sugar ingestion. It is now generally agreed that the principal dietary factor contributing to maturity-onset diabetes is an **excess of calories** relative to physical activity level.[2] A deficiency of fiber in a Western-type diet is also postulated to play a role. It has been demonstrated that a diet high in complex carbohydrate results in improved glucose tolerance with either decreased or unchanged insulin requirements.[13, 14] A Western diet high in saturated animal fat and cholesterol is probably an important contributor to macrovascular complications of diabetes due to its blood cholesterol raising effect.[2, 15] For example, Oriental diabetics on a low animal fat high starch diet have a much lower incidence of such complications.

Effect of Aging. The increase of maturity-onset diabetes appears to increase with age and the majority of diabetics in our society are over age 40.[1,2] Glucose tolerance also decreases with age. This increasing incidence of diabetes with age is probably related to the usual age-associated increase in adiposity, and decrease in physical activity in our society, however, age-induced cellular changes cannot be excluded.

Endocrine Disorders. Many hormones have metabolic actions which are counter-regulatory to those of insulin, and increases insulin requirements.[16] These include thyroid hormones, catecholamines (norepinephrine and epinephrine), cortisone, glucagon, growth hormone, and sex hormones. Thus, excesses of any of the "anti-insulin" hormones can bring about a "diabetic" metabolic state. Examples of endocrine states which precipitate diabetes include hyperthyroidism, Cushing's disease (hypercorticosteroidism) primary hyperaldosteronism, acromegaly (excess growth hormone) and pheochromocytoma (excess catecholamines). Pregnancy may also convert a prediabetic state to a temporary or permanent subclinical or manifest diabetes.[2, 3]. The incidence of diabetes also increases with multiple pregnancies.

Effects of Drugs. Medications which may produce manifest diabetes in susceptible individuals include long-term glucocorticoid steroid therapy ("steroid diabetes"), thyroid hormones, oral contraceptive agents, and thiazide or related diuretics.[3]

Pancreatic and Liver Disease. Acute and chronic pancreatitis, carcinoma of the pancreas, hemochromatosis, mucovisidosis and other diseases involving the pancreas can lead to diabetes if a significant proportion of the islet cells are destroyed.[3] Cirrhosis of the liver is associated with an increased incidence of diabetes, characterized by poor response to insulin (hepatogenic diabetes).

Effect of Stress. It has been postulated that acute or chronic emotional stress can cause diabetes through increased sympathetic nervous system stimulation and associated increased epinephrine and glucocorticoid secretions from the adrenals, however, the evidence is not decisive.[2] A transient increase in blood sugar may result from acute stress, but this is self-limited and if stress continues the response lessens due to adaptations.

CLINICAL ASPECTS OF DIABETES

Common Symptons

Laboratory Diagnosis.[3] A good laboratory is essential for diagnosis, control, and surveilance of diabetes. Commonly used tests for detecting and monitoring diabetes are listed below:

1. **Determination of Blood Sugar:** Fasting or 1 hour after a carbohydrate-rich meal.

2. **Oral Glucose Tolerance Test:** After a sample of blood is taken for fasting blood sugar, 100 g of glucose or a commercial test drink is administered and blood samples for glucose values are collected every 30 minutes for at least 120 minutes. This is useful in detecting subclinical diabetes.

3. **Glycosylated Hemoglobin:** A new laboratory test for evaluating long-term blood sugar control consists of measuring the level of glucose binding to hemoglobin ($Hb-A_1$) and is based on the observation that chronic high serum glucose levels are associated with increased non-enzymatic binding to protein.[17]

4. **Insulin Secretion:** Determination of plasma insulin levels by radio-immuno-assay[18] before and after a glucose challenge is of value in distinguishing diabetes due to insulin deficiency from the insulin resistance syndrome.

Complications

The natural history or course of diabetes is extremely variable.[19] It is difficult to predict a specific course for any given person. Many diabetics from all walks of life are able to carry on active productive lives despite severe juvenile-type diabetes, and remain free of complications. While others even under good control, appear to be plagued with complications. Diabetic complications may be classified as early or late.

Early Complications.　These are acute situations which may occur anytime in the couse of diabetes, and are usually temporary and remediable. These include the following:

1. **Diabetic Ketoacidosis or Coma.** Before the discovery of insulin, 64% died in diabetic coma, while currently only 1% die of this complication.[19]

2. **Hypoglycemia (Insulin Reaction).** Hypoglycemia or low blood sugar is one of the most common complications for diabetics, resulting from overtreatment with insulin or an oral hypoglycemic agent, from insufficient food intake to cover insulin dose, or from more physical activity than the individual customarily does.[4] Symptoms of hypoglycemia usually occur when blood sugar level drops, below 50 mg/dl; however, diabetics may experience symptoms at much higher levels in response to insulin therapy. Symptoms are of both sympathetic and central nervous system origin and include hunger, weakness, trembling, sweating, confusion, and headaches. If the diabetic doesn't respond to these prodromal symptoms by drinking a carbohydrate-rich beverage or eating carbohydrate rich foods, symptoms can progress to drowsiness or unconsciousness. Occasionally, someone with subclinical diabetes develops hypoglycemia as an initial presentation due to inappropriate timing and amounts of insulin released following meals.

Late (Long-Term) Complications[2],[4],[19]   The late complications are unlikely to occur until the diabetes has been present at least a year and increase in frequency with duration of the disease.[19] These are the main causes of premature mortality in diabetics. They usually are classified as microangiopathies (microvascular) complications; macroangiopathy (macrovascular or atherosclerotic) complications; and neuropathies. The microangiopathies and neuropathies are specific for diabetes; prevalence is less in the adult-onset type.

MICROANGIOPATHIES

Diabetic Retinopathy

This is the most common complication of diabetes and is found in one quarter to one-half of all diabetics.[20] The occurrence of microaneurysms in the area of the retinal capillaries is the characteristic lesion. The lesions may be benign and not interfere with vision. However, they can result in retinal hemorrhage, scarring and new vessel formation (proliferative retinopathy), retinal detachment and progressive visual impairment and blindness.

Diabetics also have an increased incidence of glaucoma and cataracts which also can contribute to impaired vision. Although many long-term diabetics have some degree of visual impairment, relatively few become completely blind, probably not more than 2%.[19]

Diabetic Glomerulosclerosis (Kimmelstiel-Wilson's Disease)

Kidney failure is a common cause of death in long-term juvenile diabetes, accounting for about 50% of deaths.[1],[18] It is a much less common cause of deaths in adult onset diabetes (only 6% of deaths). The initial manifestation is the finding of albumin in the urine (proteinuria). As this progresses, hypoalbuminemia occurs and results in edema. The renal lesions are associated with increases in blood pressure, blood cells and casts in the urine, a progressive rise in blood urea nitrogen and serum creatinine levels and finally, uremia. Atherosclerosis of the renal vessels and chronic pyelonephritis usually contribute to the progressive loss of renal functions.

MACROANGIOPATHY (ATHEROSCLEROSIS)

Predisposing Factors. An accelerated form of atherosclerosis leading to cardiovascular disease is common both Type I and Type II diabetes. Typically, atherosclerotic complications appear after many years of insulin-dependent diabetes, usually after microvascular disease is apparent. However, non-insulin dependent maturity-onset diabetics may present with atherosclerosis of the coronary and peripheral vessels relatively early in the course of known diabetes. This probably reflects atherosclerotic changes beginning during the subclinical phase. In the Framingham study[20], the incidence of cardiovascular disease among diabetic men was about twice that of non-diabetic men. Among diabetic women, the incidence was about three times that among non-diabetic women. About two-thirds to three quarters of all deaths in diabetics in Western societies are attibuted to cardiovascular disease.[1-4, 21]

An increased understanding of some of the reasons for accelerated atherosclerosis in diabetics is now emerging and has recently been reviewed.[2, 15, 20-23] Multiple factors appear to be involved. In particular, endothelial (artery lining) abnormalities, platelet malfunction, and lipid-lipoprotein disturbances. Possible endothelial abnormalities include premature cellular aging, altered permeability to plasma proteins and osmotic damage to the endothelium due to accumulation of an abnormal metabolite, the sugar alcohol sorbitol. Endothelial damage may be accelerated by elevated blood pressure frequently found associated with diabetes.[24] Platelet hyperaggregability and an associated diminished capacity of the body to counter-regulate against platelet deposition on damaged endothelium has also been demonstrated in diabetics. It has long been recognized that poorly controlled diabetics frequently have elevated plasma triglycerides and its principal carrier in the fasting state, very low density lipoprotein (VLDL). VLDL may be converted to a low density lipoprotein (LDL) in the artery wall, accelerating cholesterol deposition.[22] In patients with high plasma triglyceride and VLDL levels there is a predictable depression of plasma levels of high density lipoprotein (HDL)-cholesterol. Reduced HDL-cholesterol and elevated total and LDL cholesterol levels may also be found in maturity onset diabetics with normal triglyceride concentrations.[25] The resulting high total cholesterol or LDL to HDL ratio is believed to favor the deposition of cholesterol in tissues.[26] It has repeatedly been demonstrated in longitudinal epidemiologic studies that coronary heart disease patients are likely to have high total cholesterol and low HDL cholesterol levels. These lipid abnormalities are likely to be a major cause of accelerated atherlosclerosis in diabetics.[23] A low carbohydrate-high fat diet formerly favored for diabetics probably accelerates cholesterol deposition in the artery linings by raising total cholesterol and LDL levels.[2] Obesity and physical inactivity probably also contribute to an unfavorable blood lipid profile. Both are often associated with increased plasma triglycerides and VLDL and reduced HDL-cholesterol levels.

There also is evidence in the literature that high blood insulin levels (hyperinsulinemia) common in obese maturity-onset diabetics promotes the atherosclerotic process. Epidemiologic studies have shown a positive relationship of plasma insulin levels to coronary heart disease risk.[27] Furthermore, experimental studies reveal that hyperinsulinemia increases lipid synthesis and deposition in the arterial wall and proliferation of arterial smooth muscle cells.[27, 28] These cells have a great affinity for cholesterol and become the characteristic "foam cells" of the atherosclerotic lesion. Elevated levels of circulating insulin also promote liver synthesis of triglycerides and VLDL, as evidenced by a highly significant positive correlation between hyperinsulinemia and endogenous hyperglyceridemia.[25] There is also recent evidence that hyperinsulinemia promotes renal artery reabsorption of sodium and predisposes to hypertension.[29, 30]

CORONARY HEART DISEASE

Coronary heart disease is very common in diabetics and heart attacks are a major cause of death in both juvenile and adult diabetics.[1,2,19] Other forms of heart problems frequently found among diabetics are cardiac enlargement due to hypertension and diabetic cardiomyopathy both of which may terminate in congestive heart failure.

CEREBROVASCULAR DISEASE

The cerebral arteries are another common site of atherosclerosis in diabetics. Resulting cerebrovascular accidents (strokes) cause 6 and 15% of deaths in juvenile an adult-onset diabetics respectively.[19]

PERIPHERAL VASCULAR DISEASE

Atherosclerosis of peripheral arteries is frequently found in diabetics, particularly in older ones. Associated circulatory impairment may lead to gangrene and amputation of parts of the lower extremities. The prevalence of occlusive peripheral vascular disease in diabetic groups has been reported to range from 16 to 58% and gangrene at autopsy from 13 to 19%[1]. Gangrene appears to be 20 times more common in diabetics than non-diabetics.

DIABETIC NEUROPATHY (NERVE DAMAGE)

Almost any nerve pathway in the body can be affected by diabetes. Common symptoms include numbness, tingling or pain the lower extremities, muscle wasting and weakness, foot drop, absent ankle jerk reflex, gastrointestinal symptoms, difficulty in bladder emptying (due to loss of bladder muscle tone), and impotence.[3,4] The prevalence of neuropathy is higher in long-term juvenile diabetics and ranges from 5 to 52%.[1] The cause of the neuropathy is uncertain. Both microangiopathy of blood vessels supplying the nerves and metabolic dearrangements are postulated to contribute to the nerve damage.

DIABETIC MANAGEMENT

Goals

The treatment of diabetes is a lifetime affair. With modern treatment, the metabolic effects of the disease can be well regulated. The goal of treatment is to restore the patient's metabolism and lifestyle to a state as normal as possible. The therapeutic optimum is for the diabetic to have normal blood glucose levels and urine free of sugar at least most of the time, and to remain free of significant late complications. Although over the past 50 plus years, since the discovery of insulin, many thousands of diabetics have achieved great things in every walk of life, relatively few have remained free of late complications over many decades. Aside from the particular course of the disease, reasons for failure may lie with failure to adherence to therapy by the patient, inadequate instruction on the part of the physician and staff, or inadequacies in the conventional therapeutic regime. This has led to recent changes in the therapeutic approach, especially as it relates to traditional dietary advice. "Tight diabetic control" appears to be more effective in prevention of microvascular origin.[4] It is hoped that application of recent advances in understanding the atheroslcerotic process will reduce the toll of cardiovascular complications.

An earlier logo the American Diabetic Association, the triangle represents the symbolic balance between the three essential elements of diabetic control—diet, medication, and exercise. Even though the ADA has a new logo, these three modalities remain the bases for diabetic management. The role of the non-pharmacologic measures, diet and exercise will be discussed below.

Dietary Management

Diet has traditionally been the cornerstone in the treatment of diabetes.

More than one-third of all diabetics can be satisfactorily controlled with diet alone. A large proportion of maturity-onset diabetics are obese and **reduction of excess body weight often results in satisfactory regulation.**[2, 4] Thus, reduction in total calories to help in attaining ideal weight is an important goal in diabetic management. This is not a new observation since caloric restriction was the primary basis of therapy in the pre-insulin era. The importance of total calorie content in determining insulin requirements also has been known since the advent of insulin therapy.

The amount of carbohydrate to recommend for patients with diabetes has long been a subject of much debate. Until recent years, the prevailing view on diets for diabetics was that since the affected individual had elevated blood sugar levels with sugar spilling over into the urine, carbohydrates should be restricted and more calories obtained instead from proteins and fats. However, evidence has been accumulating since the 1930's that improved carbohydrate tolerance and diminished insulin requirements results from a diet high in complex carbohydrate, usually in the form of starchy, high-fiber foods. Conversely, restriction in carbohydrate intake in normal individuals produces a temporary metabolic state similar to diabetes ("starvation diabetes"). It appears from currently available data that a high carbohydrate intake improves peripheral cellular sensitivity to insulin and promotes glucose utilization.[2, 13, 14] Fiber rich meals also reduce postprandial hyperglycemia and glycosuria in insulin-dependent diabetics and may allow insulin doses to be reduced.[31] Another important concern relative to the previously traditional low carbohydrate diabetic diet is that it is high in total fat, saturated fat, and cholesterol. Such a diet has clearly been demonstrated to elevate blood lipids, and accelerate the atherosclerotic process, and thereby, likely contributes to the cardiovascular complications of diabetics. Based on the above evidence, in 1971 the American Diabetes Association's Committee on Foods recommended that "there no longer appears to be any need to restrict disproportionately the intake of carbohydrate in the diet of most diabetic patients". Enlightened current recommendations include an increase in the proportion of carbohydrate intake up to 50 to 70% of daily calories at the expense of the fat intake, which is decreased proportionately. Protein intake remains at between 15 and 20% of energy intake, but an increased amount should come from vegetable sources in place of animal sources. Most of the carbohydrate should be obtained in the form of starch from grains and starchy roots, and from fruits and vegetables. These dietary recommendations are similar to the recommended U.S. Dietary goals as proposed by the Senate Select Committee on Nutrition.[32] This liberalized dietary approach does not give diabetics a carte blanche to eat all the carbohydrate calories they want. Intake of simple sugars should be kept down as part of calories control, because they are rapidly absorbed causing widespread plasma glucose levels with hyperglycemic peaks. Salt intake should also be restricted because of the frequent association of diabetes and hypertension. It remains to be proven whether this modified diabetic diet will reduce the toll of vascular complications. Other dietary considerations include proper selection of foods to cover all nutrients needs, adequate caloric intake to satisfy usual energy expenditure and special circumstances, and stability in caloric intake and proper timing of food intake for the insulin-dependent diabetic. Generally in the latter case, the basic meal structure is three main meals plus snacks at mid-morning and mid-afternoon and at bedtime. Diet exchange systems such as used by the ADA have proven useful in training patients.[3, 4, 13] Recommended dietary goals are summarized in Table 1.

TABLE 1. Recommended Dietary Goals for Diabetics

1. If obese reduce calories to gradually obtain ideal weight.
2. Liberalize intake of complex carbohydrates.
3. Reduce intake of total fat, saturated fat, and cholesterol.
4. Avoid simple sugars.
5. Nutritionally sound meals.
6. For insulin-dependent diabetics, spread the food intake throughout the waking part of the day and keep the amount stable.

SPECIAL PROBLEMS

THE ROLE OF INCREASED PHYSICAL ACTIVITY AND AEROBIC EXERCISE

Metabolic Effects of Acute Exercise and Relationship to Diabetes

The metabolic effects of acute exercise in diabetics and their therapeutic implications has recently been extensively reviewed.[33-37] During acute exercise major metabolic, hormonal, and cardiovascular adjustments are required in order to increase the supply of fuels and oxygen to the working skeletal muscles and maintain adequate levels to vital organs. These exercise-induced changes have therapeutic value in the management of diabetes mellitus and perhaps, in prevention of cardiovascular complications. Muscle glycogen, blood-borne glucose, and free fatty acid (FFA) are the principal fuels during exercise. The relative contribution of each to oxidative energy production depends on the intensity and duration of muscular work. An orderly sequence of fuel utilization takes place during prolonged aerobic exercise, such as walking, running, cycling or swimming. During the initial phase, intramuscular glycogen is the primary source of fuel for contracting muscle. After the first 5 to 10 minutes blood glucose and FFA became increasingly important substrates. Glucose utilization during prolonged mild to moderate exercise may increase 20 times over the basal level and account for 25 to 40% of the total oxidative fuel requirements. Despite the marked stimulation of glucose utilization, blood glucose levels usually remain virtually unchanged or only slightly decrease during the first 40 minutes of exercise. This is because the blood glucose pool is continuously augmented by an increase in glucose released from the liver (three to fivefold). For the first 40 minutes, most of liver glucose production (about 75%) is derived from breakdown of hepatic glycogen (glycogenolysis). However, such stores are limited. During more prolonged exercise formation of hepatic glycogen from various precursors (lactate, pyruvate, glycerol, and certain amino acids), i.e., **gluconeogenesis,** becomes increasing important and may account for 40 to 50% of hepatic glucose output. Eventually, if exercise is continued long enough, blood glucose levels begin to fall despite gluconeogenesis. A progressive shift in energy metabolism from carbohydrate to FFA occurs and the FFA contribution to oxidative metabolism may be twice that of glucose. A direct relationship exists between levels of plasma FFA and muscle utilization. Following exercise, the exercise-induced fall in glycogen content of the working muscle induces prolonged stimulation of glycogen synthetase for glycogen resynthesis, and leads to prolonged increased glucose uptake.[37],[38] Replenishment of muscle and liver glycogen stores takes about 24 to 48 hours. During this period, there is an improvement in glucose tolerance and dimished insulin requirements.

A variety of hormonal changes are involved in the regulation of fuel availability, utilization, and homeostasis during exercise. The essential role of insulin in glucose utilization during exercise is illustrated by studies in depancreatized dogs in whom exercise did not increase glucose utilization until small doses of replacement insulin were given.[39] However, with prolonged exercise there is a fall in plasma insulin levels in proportion to duration of exercise. Reduction in plasma levels may persist for several days after exercise. This is related at least in part in untrained subjects to an increased cellular receptor affinity to insulin.[11],[40] Reduced circulating insulin levels contributes to stimulation of glucose production by the liver and to FFA mobilization from adipose tissue. Increased secretion of several so-called counter-regulatory hormones is related to both intensity and duration of exercise. During exercise the plasma levels of these hormones, in particular catecholamines glucagon, growth hormone, and cortisol, become elevated. All of them contribute to hepatic glucose production and FFA mobilization from adipose tissue.

In insulin-dependent diabetes the metabolic response to exercise is largely determined by adequacy of diabetic control with exogenous insulin. When diabetic control is adequate or if there is only mild hyperglycemia without ketosis, exercise results in reduction in blood glucose levels and insulin requirements.[33-37] Several mechanisms appear to be involved. Enhanced delivery from injection sites has been demonstrated during exercise, particularly if the exercising legs are used for insulin administration.[41] If the exercise is carried out at the peak effect of insulin administration the decline in blood glucose level may be due primarily to enhanced glucose utilization, and insulin suppression of the compensatory increase in hepatic glucose production. Thus in the usual clinical situation of adequate insulin replacement, acute exercise exerts beneficial effect on diabetic control by reducing hyperglycemia.

In contrast, when insulin deficiency is more severe and there is associated poor metabolic control, the production of glucose, FFA, and ketone bodies may exceed peripheral utilization, thereby increasing hyperglycemia and ketoacidosis and thereby, worsening the diabetic state.[33 37] An exaggerated rise in plasma catecholamines and growth hormone may contribute, and can be normalized by better control.[40] These findings indicate the importance of adequate diabetic control prior to diabetic patients starting an exercise program.

A well-recognized potential problem in insulin-treated diabetic patients is exercise-induced hypoglycemia. The use of non-exercised injection sites for insulin, particularly the abdominal wall, reduces risk of hypoglycemia.[41] Reduction in insulin dose, avoidance of exercise at the time of peak insulin effect, exercising at the time of the usual appearance of mild glycouria, or a carbohydrate snack about ½ hour before exercising and during prolonged exercise may also help reduce the chances for hypoglycemia.[4]

Benefits of Regular Aerobic Exercise (Training or Conditioning)

Improved Diabetic Control. The beneficial effects of exercise in diabetic control were known in the pre-insulin era. Allen[42] first reported that exercise lowered blood sugar in patients with mild or moderate diabetes and could improve tolerance to a carbohydrate load. It also has been known for the past 45 years that regular exercise decreases insulin requirements in insulin dependent diabetics.[43] Exercise training likewise reduces insulin secretion in response to a glucose challenge in non-insulin dependent diabetics as well as non-diabetics.[33] [37] [44] [47]

Repeated regular exercise potentiates the acute metabolic and hormonal adaptations accompanying acute exercise, which no doubt contributes to reduced insulin requirements. Recent studies have demonstrated that exercise training also increases cellular sensitivity to insulin in both diabetics and non-diabetics by significantly increasing numbers of insulin receptors in proportion to improvement in physical fitness.[10–12, 40] This is especially important in management of the insulin resistance syndrome associated with obesity and maturity-onset diabetes. Reduced secretion of anti-insulin hormones such as catecholamines and glucagon after training may also enhance diabetic control.

Correction or Prevention of Obesity. The role of obesity in insulin resistance and etiology of maturity-onset diabetes was previously discussed. Physical inactivity is often a major contributor to obesity in modern society. Regular exercise can reduce chances for diabetes by helping weight maintenance in addition to the direct metabolic and endocrine adaptations discussed above. The value of regular walking exercise in normalizing body weight and mobilizing adipose stores in obese people in the absence of dietary changes recently has been demonstrated.[46, 48] The loss of lean body mass during weight reduction associated with caloric restriction is not observed when exercise is used alone or in combination with moderate caloric restriction in a weight reduction program.[46, 49] Weight loss through exercise may exceed that which would be anticipated through direct expenditure of calories.[46] Two likely processes are believed to play a role: (1) appetite suppression and (2) a persistent increase in resting metabolic rate following exercise.

Skeletal Muscle Adaptations.[50, 51] Skeletal muscle converts chemical energy into mechanical energy to make contraction and physical mobility possible. Training improves muscle tone and strength and increases capillary blood supply to each muscle fiber. This results in improved delivery and extraction of oxygen and nutrient substrates. Increase in muscle content of the oxygen binding pigment, myoglobin contributes to improved oxygen uptake. Glycogen storage capacity is also markedly increased. In addition, an increase in muscle oxidative metabolic capacity results from an augmentation in numbers of mitochondria and in a substantial increase in their contained oxidative and respiratory chain enzymes. These adaptations markedly increase utilization by the trained muscle during exercise of glucose, FFA, and ketone bodies with less lactic acid production. Thus training effects on skeletal muscle can make significant contributions to control of diabetes as well as improving work capacity.

Effect on Blood Lipids and Lipoproteins. Exercise training may reduce lipid abnormalities frequently associated with diabetes. A decrease in elevated levels of plasma triglycerides and their principal carrier in the fasting state VLDL has been demonstrated in both non-diabetics and maturity-onset diabetics.[36, 52, 53] An increased breakdown and utilization of triglycerides as a fuel during exercise is potentiated with training by increased activity of lipoprotein lipasse in muscle and adipose tissue.[36] Decreased hepatic synthesis of triglycerides in response to reduced circulating insulin probably contributes. Effects of training on plasma total cholesterol levels in non-diabetics and diabetics are variable. Several groups have reported a decrease and others no change.[36] Increased levels of HDL cholesterol have been observed with training in young and middle-aged and non-diabetic men.[46, 54] However, recent controlled dietary studies indicate that this change in non-diabetics is probably primarily due to associated weight loss.[55, 56] We also failed to find any significant change in HDL cholesterol with brisk walking for up to 60 minutes four times per week for 12 weeks in maturity-onset diabetics in whom weight was held constant.[47] Improved diabetic control alone is reported to raise HDL cholesterol levels.[57, 58] Since an inverse relationship exists between plasma HDL cholesterol levels and premature coronary heart disease, increased levels should help protect diabetics against this common vascular complication.

Reduced Risk of Coronary Heart Disease. An inverse relationship between physical activity levels and incidence of coronary heart disease and associated mortality has repeatedly been demonstrated in epidemiologic studies.[51, 59] Optimal protection appears to be afforded by 2,000 kcal per week of physical activity and partial protection by at least 500 kcal per week.[60] Possible physiological mechanisms by which exercise reduces coronary risk include the blood lipid changes described above, reduced circulating insulin levels, improved glucose tolerance, lower body weight, reduced blood pressure and heart rate, decreased myocardial oxygen requirements (as a result of decreased systolic blood pressure and heart rate), increased myocardial vascularity, reduced blood coagulability, and decreased vulnerability to serious cardiac rhythm disturbances.[51, 59] A definitive clinical trial proving the protective effects of regular exercise against coronary heart disease has not been done in either non-diabetics or diabetics; however, the available evidence is sufficient to include exercise as part of a coronary prevention program for both.

Increased Work Capacity and Endurance. One of the easiest to demonstrate benefits of exercise training in both diabetics and non-diabetics is enhanced cardio-respiratory endurance as measured by increased maximal oxygen uptake. This usually results from improvement in both stroke volume of the heart and increased arterialvenous oxygen difference. The functional value of this training effect is an increase in maximal work capacity and the ability to perform sub-maximal work longer with less perceived effort and fatigue.

Psychosocial Benefits. Physical activity results in a variety of psychosocial benefits which improve quality of life. Activities should be selected which are fun and enjoyable to the individual. The resulting improved feeling of well-being, health consciousness, self-confidence, self-control, self-esteem are especially important for patients with a chronic disease such as diabetes.[4] Exercise is also helpful in relieving muscular tension and mental depression, and it promotes sound sleep.[61]

Principles for Increasing Physical Activity and Fitness

Activities should be selected which the individual enjoys, are appropriate for his or her health and fitness level, and can be maintained for a lifetime. They should involve rhythmic movements of the large muscle groups of the body and be of mild to moderate intensity and non-exhausting (in other words, isonic, aerobic activities). It is helpful in order to properly adjust food intake and medications if the activities of insulin-dependent diabetics can be quantitated. Examples of ideal activities for diabetic management include walking, hiking, slow running (jogging), swimming, bicycling, and cross-country skiing. Such activities will significantly improve aerobic capacity (maximal oxygen uptake) and provide other physiologic and psychologic benefits previously described if performed regularly (at least 3 to 5 days per week) for an hour at a time at a moderate level of intensity (60% of maximal oxygen uptake or 70% of maximal heart rate).[62] To obtain optimal levels for coronary protection according to Paffenbarger et al,[60] one would need to walk about 3 miles or about an hour on a daily basis. Diabetics should also take advantage of opportunities around them in their work or home environment to expend more energy. This could include walking or bicycling instead of driving to work, walking briskly from a distant parking lot, climbing stairs instead of elevators, walking around the work environment during coffee and lunch breaks, standing instead of sitting whenever possible, cleaning house, washing and maintaining the car, gardening, walking the dog, dancing, and avoiding labor saving devices such as power lawn mowers and snow blowers.

Exercise Precautions and Guidelines (Table II)

The diabetic should understand both the benefits and possible adverse effects of exercise. The need to avoid strenuous exercise until reasonable diabetic control is established was previously discussed. For the insulin-dependent diabetic, the principal risk is insulin reaction or hypoglycemia. This necessitates a regular pattern of exercise. Exercise should be performed at the same convenient time every day at approximately the same intensity and duration. It is best that exercise not be performed at the time of peak insulin effect, however, this can be compensated for by a carbohydrate snack about half an hour before exercising. Because of the pro-insulin effect of exercise, the insulin-dependent diabetic upon initiating an exercise program will have to reduce insulin dose or increase food intake. Insulin dosage usually has to be reduced 20% or more. The need to avoid administration of insulin to sites on exercising limbs was previously discussed. During prolonged activities, a 10 gm. carbohydrate snack, (fruit, fruit juice, or soft drink) is recommended for each 30 minutes of activity. Activities should be stopped at initial warning symptoms of hypoglycemia and an carbohydrate snack or beverage taken. It is also a good idea that the diabetic not exercise alone and make certain that his or her partner is aware of the possibility of a hypoglycemic reaction. Adequate fluid replacement during and after exercise is important to avoid dehydration.

Good footware and careful foot hygiene are extremely important to the diabetic to avoid injuries, corns, blisters, and other foot problems which may lead to serious complications because of frequent association of peripheral vascular disease, neuropathy, and tendency for infections.

Before diabetic individuals embark on any exercise program, more strenuous than brisk walking, a careful medical evaluation is necessary to rule out contraindications and to prescribe safe levels of exercise. A multistage exercise electrocardiogram test should be included to rule out manifestations of significant latent coronary artery disease and to establish a baseline fitness level. The prescribed exercise should be commensurate with the severity of diabetes, fitness status, and recreational interests of the individual and availability of facilities. In order to minimize risk of musculoskeletal problems, the initial starting level of programs should be short duration and gradually progress. A warm-up and cool-down period should be included. Generally for the middle-aged or older diabetic, competitive and isometric activities should be avoided because of the possibility of excessive cardiovascular stress.

TABLE 2. Exercise Dangers and Preventive Measures

1. Aggrevation of Diabetic Metabolic Dearrangements
   a. Avoid strenuous exercise until diabetes is controlled.
   b. Adequate fluid replacement.

2. Exercise-induced Hypoglycemia (Insulin-Dependent Diabetics)
   a. Insulin administration to abdominal wall.
   b. Reduce insulin dosage and/or increase food intake.
   c. Avoid exercise during peak insulin activity.
   d. Carbohydrate snacks before and during prolonged exercise.
   e. Reproducible regular exercise.
   f. Prompt recognition and response to symptoms.
   g. Knowledgeable companion along.

2. Foot problems
   a. Proper footwear.
   b. Foot hygiene.

4. Cardiovascular Complications
   a. Pre-exercise medical evaluation.
   b. Exercise ECG test.
   c. Individualized exercise prescription.
   d. Avoid competitive activities.

5. Musculo-Skeletal Injuries
   a. Appropriate selection of activities.
   b. Start slowly and progress gradually.
   c. Warmup and cool-down.
   d. Don't overdo it.

REFERENCES

1. USDHEW: **Disabetes Data Compiled 1977.** DHEW Publication No. (NIH) 78-1468, Washington, D.C., U.S. Gov't Printing Office, 1978.

2. West, K.M.: **Epidemiology of Diabetes and Its Vascular Lesions.** New York, Elsevier-North Holland, Inc., 1978.

3. Petrides, P., Weiss, L., Loffler, G., and Wieland, O.H.: **Diabetes Mellitus: Theory and Management.** Baltimore-Munich, Urban & Schwarzenberg, 1978,

4. Krall, L.P.: **Joslin Diabetic Manual.** 11th Edition. Philadelphia, Lea & Febiger, 1978.

5. West, K.M.: Standardization of definition, classification, and reporting in diabetes-related epidemiologic studies. **Diabetes Care,** 2:65-76, 1979.

6. Rotter, J.I. and Rimon, D.L.. Diabetes mellitus: The search for genetic markers. **Diabetic Care,** 2:215-226, 1979.

7. Berger, M., Muller, W.A., and Renold, A.E.: Relationship of obesity to obesity: Some facts, many questions. **In Diabetes, Obesity, and Vascular Disease.** Edited by H.M. Katzen and R.J. Mahler. New York, John Wiley & Sons, 1978, Part 1: 211-222.

8. Reaven, G.M. and Olefsky, J.M.: Role of insulin resistance in the pathogenesis of hyperglycemia. **In Diabetes, Obesity and Vascular Disease.** Edited by H.M. Katzen and R.J. Mahler. New York, John Wiley & Sons, 1978, Part I: 229-260.

9. Lipman, R.L., Raskin, P., Love, T., Triebwasser, J., Lecocq, F.R. and Schure, J.J.: Glucose tolerance during decreased physical activity in man. **Diabetes,** 21:101-107, 1972.

10. Pedersen, O., Beck-Neilsen, H., and Heding, L.: Increased insulin receptors after exercise in patients with insulin-dependent diabetes mellitus. **N. Engl. J. Med.,** 302:886-892, 1980.

11. Soman, V.R., Koivosto, V.A., Diebert, D., Felig, P., and DeFronzo, R.A..

Increased insulin sensitivity and insulin binding to monocytes after physical training. **N. Engl. J. Med.,** 301:1200-1204, 1979.

12. Koivisto, V.A., Soman, V., Conrad, P., Hendler, R., Nadel, E., and Felig, P.: Insulin binding to monocytes in trained athletes. Changes in the resting state and after exercise. **Am. Soc. Clin. Invest.,** 64:1011-1015, 1979.

13. Skyler, J.S.: Nutritional management of diabetes mellitus. **In Diabetes, Obesity, and Vascular Disease.** Edited by H.M. Katzen and R.J. Mahler. New York, John Wiley & Sons, 1978, Part 2: 645-686.

14. Feldman, J.M.: Diet in diabetic patients with heart disease. **In Diabetes and the Heart.** Edited by S. Zoneraich. Springfield, Charles C. Thomas, 1978, 238-258.

15. Bierman, E.L. and Brunzell, J.D.: Interrelation of atherosclerosis, abnormal lipid metabolism, and diabetes mellitus. **In Diabetes, Obesity, and Vascular Disease.** Edited by H.M. Katzen and R.J. Mahler. New York, John Wiley & Sons, 1978, Part 1: 187-207.

16. Eaton, R.P. and Schabe, D.S.: Modulation and implications of the counter-regulatory hormones: glucagon, catecholamines, cortisol, and growth hormone. **In Diabetes, Obesity, and Vascular Disease.** Edited by H.M. Katzen and R.J. Mahler. New York, John Wiley & Sons, 1978, Part 1: 341-366.

17. Bunn, H.F., Gabbay, K.H., and Gallop, P.M.: The gycosylation of hemoglobin relevance to diabetes mellitus. **Science,** 200:21-27, 1978.

18. Hales, C.N. and Randle, P.J.: Immunoassay of insulin with insulin antibody precipitate. **Biochem. J.,** 88:737-746, 1973.

19. Davidson, M.B.: The continuing changing natural history of diabetes. **J. Chronic Dis.,** 34:5-10, 1918.

20. Kannel, W.B. and McGee, D.L.: Diabetes and cardiovascular disease: The Framingham Study. **JAMA,** 241:2035-2038, 1979.

21. Knowles, H.C., Jr.: Coronary artery disease in diabetes: Its development, course, and response to treatment. **In Diabetes and the Heart.** Edited by S. Zoneraich Springfield, Charles C. Thomas, 1978, 113-122.

22. Spritz, N.: Diabetes, Heart Disease and Hyperlipidemia. **In Diabetes and the Heart.** Edited by S. Zoneraich. Springfield, Charles C. Thomas, 1978, 137-143.

23. Colwell, J.A.: Atherosclerosis in diabetes mellitus. **J. Chronic Dis.,** 34:1-4, 1981.

24. Christlieb, A.R.: Hypertension, diabetes and the heart. **In Diabetes and the Heart.** Edited by S. Zoneraich. Springfield, Charles C. Thomas, 1978, 175-192.

25. Saudek, C.D. and Eder, H.A.: Lipid metabolism in diabetes mellitus. **Am. J. Med.,** 66:843-852, 1979.

26. Miller, G. and Miller, N.E.: Plasma high density lipoprotein concentration and development of ischemic heart disease. **Lancet,** 1:16-19, 1975.

27. Pyorala, K.: Relationship of glucose tolerance and plasma insulin to the incidence of coronary heart disease: Results from two population studies in Finland. **Diabetes Care,** 2:131-141, 1979.

28. Stout, R.W.: **The relationship of abnormal circulatory insulin levels to atherosclerosis. Arteriosclerosis,** 27:1-13, 1977.

29. Sims, E.A.H.: Mechanisms of hypertension in the syndrome of obesity. **Intern. J. Obesity,** 5(Supple 1):9-18, 1981.

30. Horton, E.S. The role of exercise in the treatment of hypertension in obesity. **Intern. J. Obesity,** 5(Supple. 1):165-171, 1981.

31. Anderson, J.W. and Chen, W-J.L.: Plant fiber, carbohydrate and lipid metabolism. **Am. J. Clin. Nutr.,** 32:346-363, 1979.

32. Select Committee on Nutrition and Human Needs, **U.S. Senate Dietary Goals for the United States,** 2nd Ed., Washington, D.C., U.S. Govt. Printing Office.

33. Felig, P. and Koivisto, V.A.: The metabolic response to exercise: Implications for diabetes. **In Therapeutics Through Exercise.** Editied by D.T. Lowenthal, K. Bharadwaja, and W.W. Oaks. New York, Grune and Stratton, 1979, 3-20.

34. Wahren, J., Felig, P. and Hagenfeldt, L: Physical exercise and fuel

homeostasis in diabetes mellitus. **Diabetologia,** 14:213-222, 1978.

35. Vranic, M. and Berger, M.: Exercise and diabetes mellitus. **Diabetes,** 28:147-163, 1979.

36. Koivisto, V.A. and Sherwin, R.S.: Exercise in diabetes. Therapeutic implications. **Postgrad. Med.,** 66:87-96, 1979.

37. Richter, E.A. and Ruderman, N.B.: Diabetes and exercise. **Am.J.Med.,** 70:201-209, 1981.

38. Wahren, J.: Glucose turnover during exercise in healthy man and in patients with diabetes mellitus. **Diabetes,** 28 (Suppl. 1):82-88, 1979.

39. Berger, M., Hagg, S., and Ruderman, N.B.: Glucose metabolism in perfused skeletal muscle. Interaction of insulin and exercise on glucose uptake. **Biochem. J.,** 146:231-38, 1975.

40. Koivisto, V.A., Soman, V., Nadel, E., Tamborlane, W.V., and Felig, P.: Exercise and insulin: insulin binding, insulin mobilization, and counterregulatory hormone secretion. **Fed.Proc.,** 39:1481-1486, 1980.

41. Zinman, B., Vranic, M., Albisser., A.M., Liebel, B.S. and Marliss, E.B.: The role of insulin in the metabolic response to exercise in diabetic men. **Diabetes,** 28 (Suppl. 1):76-81, 1979.

42. Allen, F.M.: Notes concerning exercise in the treatment of severe diabetes. Boston, **Med.Surg.J.,** 173:743-744, 1915.

43. Lawrence, R.D.: Effects of exercise on insulin action in diabetes. **Brit. Med. J.,** 1:648,650, 1926.

44. Saltin, B., Lindgarde, F., Houston, M., Horlin, R., Nygard, E. and Gad, P.: Physical training and glucose tolerance in middle-aged men with chemical diabetes. **Diabetes,** 28, (Suppl 1) :30-39, 1979.

45. Bjorntorp, P.: Effect of exercise and physical training and carbohydrate and lipid metabolism in man. **Adv. Cardiol.,** 18:158-166, 1976.

46. Leon, A.S., Conrad, J.C., Hunninghake, D.B., and Serfass, R.: Effect of a vigorous walking program on body composition and carbohydrate and lipid metabolism on obese young men. **Am.J.Clin. Nutri.,** 33:1776-1787, 1979.

47. Leon, A.S., Conrad, J.C., Casal, D.C., and Goetz, F.: Failure of diabetes

alone to control maturity-onset diabetes (abstr.). **Med.Sci.Sports,** 12:104, 1980.

48. Gwinup, G.: Effect of exercise alone on weight of obese women. **Arch.Int.Med.,** 135:675-680, 1975.

49. Brownell, K.D. and Stunkard, A.J.: Physical activity in the development of control of obesity. **In Obesity.** Edited by A.J. Stunkard. Philadelphia, W.B. Saunders, 1980, 300-324.

50. Holloszy, J.O., Rennie, M.J., Hickson, R.C., Conolee, R.K., and Hagberg, J.M.: Physiological consequences of the biochemical adaptation to endurance exercise. **Ann. NY Acad.Sci.,** 301:440-454, 1977.

51. Winder, W.W.: Adaptation of skeletal muscle to exercise. **In Therapeutics Through Exercise.** Edited by D.T. Lowenthal, K. Bharadwaja, and W.W. Oaks. New York, Grune and Stratton, 1979, 33-40.

52. Wyndham, C.H.: The role of physical activity in the prevention of ischemic heart disease. A review. **SA Med.J.,** 56:7-13, 1979.

53. Ruderman, N.B., Granada, O.P., and Johanson, K.: The effect of physical training on glucose tolerance and plasma lipids in maturity-onset diabetes. **Diabetes,** 28 (Suppl 1):89-92, 1979.

54. Hartung, G.H., Squires, W.G., and Gotto, A.M.: Effect of exercise training on plasma high-density lipoprotein cholesterol in coronary heart patients. **Am.Heart J.,** 101:181-184, 1981.

55. Lipson, L.C., Bonow, R.O., Schaefer, E.J., Brewer, E.J. and Lindgren, F.T.: Effect of exercise conditioning on plasma high density lipoproteins and other lipoproteins. **Artherosclerosis,** 37:529-538, 1980.

56. Leon, A.S. and Sopko, G.: Unpublished data, 1981.

57. Calvert, G.D., Mannik, T., Graham, J.J., Wise, P.H., and Yeates, R.A.: Effects of therapy on plasma-high-density-lipoprotein concentration in diabetes mellitus. **Lancet,** 2:66-68, 1978.

58. Lopes-Virella, M.F.L., Stone, P.G. and Colwell, J.A.: Serum high density

lipoprotein in diabetes patients. **Diabetologia,** 13:285-291, 1977.

59. Leon, A.S. and Blackburn, H.: The relationship of physical activity to coronary heart disease and life expectancy. **Ann. NY Acad.Sci.,** 301:656-568, 1977.

60. Paffenbarger, R.S., Jr., Wing, A.L., and Hyde, R.T.: Physical activity as an index of heart attack risk in college alumni. **Am.J. Epidemiol.** 108:161-175, 1978.

61. Folkins, C.H., and Amsterdam, E.A.: Control and modification of stress emotions through chronic exercise. **In Exercise in Cardiovascular Health and Disease.** Edited by E.A. Amsterdam, J.H. Wilmore, and A.N. DeMars. New York, Yorke Medical Books, 1977, 280-294.

62. Pollock, M.L.: How much exercise is enough? **Physician Sportsmed.,** 26:50-64, 1978.

Nutrition Advice For The Young Athlete

NATHAN J. SMITH, M.D.

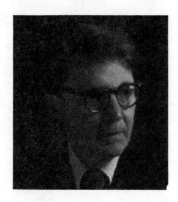

Professor of Pediatrics and Orthopedics, Division of Sports Medicine, University of Washington, Seattle.
Author of **Food for Sport, Handbook for the Young Athlete,** and numerous other books and articles regarding nutrition and athletics. Consultant to American Board of Pediatrics and on editorial board of Pediatrics In Review.

There is a distinct pyramid in the number of participants in highly organized sports in this country[1]. There are a relatively few highly competent, well-paid, professional athletes[2] at the top of this pyramid and at its base there are some twenty-million elementary and junior high school aged young people[3] actively involved in organized competitive sports, in addition to a few hundred thousand collegiate athletes at colleges and universities[4]. There are more than seven-million high school boys and girls actively competing in interscholastic sports[5]. Sports programs are expanding both in the number of sports available to students at the high school level and in the numbers of young people taking part. In almost every community there will be some sport that is participated in by almost every young person in that community. Athletic competition now begins at a very early age and has become a very important part of growing up for most children and their families.

Even though the new forms of organized play for the youth of the country are known to present certain problems, the active exercise and physical activity of training and competition are providing many physical and psycho-social benefits for both boys and girls. Actually, planned

SPECIAL PROBLEMS

energy expenditures are essential for health and fitness for those living in restricting urban environments[6]. A benefit pertinent to the concerns of this conference is the motivation of young people that sports participation creates to an increased level of concern about their diet and nutrition practices. Eating better to perform better on the court or athletic field is a concern in the mind of the athletes. The motivation for improved nutrition can provide a truly effective opportunity for sound nutrition education. There is, therefore, a responsibility for the coach, trainer and sports medicine professional to provide valid nutrition information to the athlete.

One potential problem can be identified that deserves specific attention in relation to the sport nutrition concerns of the prepubertal athlete of elementary age. The millions of young athletes of this age should be having the nutrition needs of growing up met optimally at family meal times without regard for their sport participation. The sound nutrition practices of the family of the ten year old shouldn't be based on what will make him or her a better soccer player, but rather on what will contribute to making the young person a happy and healthy eleven year old.

The one nutrition-related problem area in youth sports programs is the prepubescent's limited ability to efficiently adapt to exercising in warm environments[2]. Because the young child athlete is often put into situations where repeated training sessions and competition may take place in the heat, it is important that volunteer coaches and parents know that the prepubescent child is less efficient in thermo regulation than is the post-pubescent athlete or adult. The body's principle cooling mechanism is the evaporation of sweat from skin surfaces. The pre-pubertal child athlete is incapable of producing sweat effectively which becomes an important handicap when exercising in the heat. The prepubertal athlete does not have the ability to produce a more abundant and more diluted sweat with repeated training in the heat. These handicaps of adjustment to thermo regulation are compounded by the fact that the young athlete develops a sense of well-being more rapidly than the older athlete when exercising in the heat. Thus, with limited physiologic adjustments, the psychologic adjustments to exercise in warm environments are made more rapidly, placing the young athlete at increased risk to heat stroke or heat-induced collapse. Exercise and training in the heat must be carefully supervised, with particular attention given to maintaining adequate levels of hydration.

Many pediatricians and child health professionals are concerned about the tremendous expansion of the many community-based, youth sport activities. There is, however, quite universal enthusiasm for the increased participation in sports by young people at the high school level, especially the large number of girls now active in sports[3]. One reason is the impact on nutrition fitness of such active participation. Nutrition evaluations of high school populations, as well as more recent national nutrition surveys, clearly documented that the segment of the population at greatesk risk to unmet nutritional needs in the U.S. has been adolescents of high school age. That increased energy expenditure through sports participation would lead to increased total food intake and an increased intake of essential nutrients could be projected as a very positive consequence of a more active lifestyle.

Nutrition surveys such as the Ten State Nutrition Survey of the early seventies and the HANES that have followed have identified the national nutrition problems of a public health concern existent in our affluent food-excess society[4]. These problems are primarily concerned with maintenance of energy balances. Significant numbers of individuals fail to satisfy their normal energy demands by either voluntary or involuntary restriction of caloric intakes. Approximately fifteen percent of Americans are in the latter catagory being unable to meet their needs for food because of inadequate incomes. Large numbers of middle and upper income women voluntarily restrict their food intakes in the absence of a significant physical energy expenditure in order to avoid the unacceptable consequences of obesity. Most common of the problems of energy imbalances, of course, is the intake of food energy in excess of energy expenditure and the unavoidable result of obesity. This is a problem concentrated in populations of upper income males and low income, inactive females. The problem of specific nutrient deficiency, the concern of early nutrition surveys, is strikingly absent in the United States today; even in the poverty population of this country. With the exception of iron deficiency there is an impressive absence of either biochemical or clinical evidence of specific nutrient deficiency in the population of the United States. The dietary deficiency in the poor in this country is a quantitative one, and not a problem of the quality of the diet. Poor people in the United States eat the same good quality diet as middle and upper income individuals, but for obvious economic reasons they have less of it available to them.

As the national nutrition problems that have been so well documented during the past decade have centered around energy balance and meeting energy needs, the problems that can be most commonly identified among a population of young athletes are likewise problems concerned with satisfying energy demands[5]. The athlete in training with unusually large energy requirements may often fail to satisfy these energy demands and under perform because of lack of an adequate supply of food energy. The young high school boy or girl coming from a poverty family may have inadequate food available in the home to meet the demands of training and adolescent growth. The more affluent but disorganized family may not provide food enough to meet the high nutrition energy needs of a growing teen-aged boy in an active sports program. The over-committed student with academic, social, as well as athletic commitments, may "not have time to eat." In addition, there may be the student so immature and dependent that as a high school student, or college athlete, he or she cannot give an appropriate priority to their nutritional needs. In total, these groups make up a sizeable population of underfed, undernourished athletes, commonly encountered in any scholastic or collegiate sports programs, and because of lack of energy they perform poorly. When the young athlete under performs, first be certain that he or she is getting enough to eat.

Fortunately, it is not difficult to monitor the adequacy of total food energy intake of the active young athlete or athletic team. If the demands of training and competition exceed the athlete's energy intake, there will inevitably be unintentional weight loss. Body tissues are metabolized to satisfy the energy demands not met by food energy intakes. There will be an inevitable deterioration of performance as body weight is lost. Thus, it is important to monitor the adequacy of energy intake by scheduled and recorded nude weight two or three times weekly, at the same time on the same day of the week. Any unintentional weight loss must be readily explained and should usually be referred for medical consultation. Unexplained, unintentional weight loss is always evidence of serious organic disease until proven otherwise.

There are frequent concerns on the part of young athletes and their coaches as to whether the athletes' diets are providing an adequate intake of all the many nutrients that are known to be essential components of a desired diet. Nutrition science has identified more than fifty substances that are recognized as essential nutrients. It is important for all of those involved in sports to know that the vigorous exercise of athletic training does not significantly increase the body's need for any specific nutrient. The most actively training athlete will only have an increased need for food energy to supply the energy expended in training activities and an increased need for water to replace the water lost primarily through sweating. The athlete's need for essential nutrients is not significantly greater than that of less active individuals[6].

A simple and practical diet evaluation system developed for the assessment of the adequacy of the normal diet is appropriate for judging the adequacy of the athlete's diet. Most young athletes have had some orientation to the Four Food Group System of dietary scoring in their school experience and probably have little motivation to apply it to their personal diets until they have become involved in a competitive sport program. Nutrition scientists now know that if an individual has two servings of milk products, two servings of high protein foods such as poultry, fish, meat or beans, four servings of vegetables or fruits, and four servings of grain foods, such as bread, rolls or pastas that such a diet will provide an adequate intake of all of the essential nutrients needed for the optimal nutritional health of a healthy individual regardless of his or her level of physical activity. It is thus very helpful for a concerned young athlete to evaluate their diet by simply writing down each food item eaten during a period of a few days, review the record and determine whether there is the desired daily representation of the various food groups. This review will indicate whether some diet modification is needed. Most young athletes will be pleasantly surprised to find that a cheeseburger with lettuce and tomatoes, or a lunch of good pizza, will include the desired representation of all four of the food groups in a single preference food item.

There is one exception to the rule that the Four Food Group diet will meet the need for all essential nutrients. That exception involves the intake of iron for as many as fifteen to twenty percent of healthy females experiencing normal, but greater than average menstrual iron losses[7]. The low concentration of iron in even a high quality American diet is such that this relatively large number of women cannot meet their iron needs even though eating a high quality diet. This is the one segment of the healthy United States population where a nutritional supplement is appropriate.

Recent laboratory study has demonstrated that exercise performance is reduced in the presence of what have been thought to be mild degrees of iron deficiency[8]. These are degrees of iron deficiency where no detectable anemia is present. Athletic performance of these iron deficient athletes is definitely limited. It is therefore suggested that young girls have a biochemical assessment of their iron status early in their high school years This is especially true if they are trying to be competitive in a sport program. Iron deficiency that will limit endurance performance is also encountered among rapidly growing teen-aged boys in deprived circumstances with limited access to food. The levels of iron deficiency now documented to have performance implications forms a relatively new nutrition concern and will be commanding increasing attention in the near future. It is now important that there be developed practical and economic means for identifying the otherwise healthy, well nourished young person with a greater than average need for iron that is not being satisfied with a conventional good diet and who will need a regular medicinal iron supplement.

A prominent nutrition concern is encountered among those young athletes who are faced with the desire of need to modify their body composition to improve their performance potential in various sports. Many individuals desire to either increase muscle weight and body weight, or recognize the need to minimize body fatness and reduce body weight[9]. Elsewhere in this conference the problems of controlling fatness and body weight have been discussed in relation to weight matched competitions such as wrestling. There are other sports where even more attention may be directed to controlling the diet as fatness must be minimized for a sport in which the training activities, although occupying prolonged periods each day, result in relatively little energy expenditure. Training programs in girl's gymnastics and figure skating, present these problems. Although it is essential to establish a well planned diet, properly representing the various food groups, particular emphasis must be placed on increasing energy expenditure through regular physical exercise. This must be in addition to the activities involved in the low energy expending training schedule. Telling the young girl gymnast with a fatness problem, who is spending five or six hours a day training in her gym, that she has to now begin to get some exercise, is a message that must be delivered with some tact and discretion. It is the critical message in weight control for these young ladies nevertheless.

The single most common nutrition related concern encountered among young athletes is the nutrition advice that is sought by those desiring to increase body weight and strength to increase their playing potential in any one of many sports. Interviews with forty-eight varsity basketball players from four Seattle high schools revealed that sixty-five percent of them had tried to put on weight at some time during their high school sports careers through the use of special diets, drugs, supplements, protein powders,etc. Whether the athlete wishes to increase this weight in order to increase his playing potential for basketball, football or to be a more effective defense man on the hockey team he must first realize that only by increasing his body weight through an increase in muscle mass, will he increase his potential as an athlete. (Sumo wrestling may be one exception.) Increasing body fatness will only reduce speed and endurance and increase the risk of injury. Secondly, the athlete and the coach must recognize that only muscle work will increase muscle size and muscle weight. There is no specific nutrient, protein compound, hormone or drug, that will increase muscle mass. Thus, the athlete who wishes to increase muscle mass, strength and endurance will first schedule himself for a well supervised program of weight training. This muscle work must be participated in regularly for a period of many months of off season training. He must increase his well planned and regularly taken diet by approximately one thousand calories each day. This involves adding a fourth meal to a conventional three meal a day eating plan. Food choices are of little concern and can include any attractive selection of preferred food which can supplement the basic Four Food Group Diet. An increased food energy intake is the critical dietary contribution that will support the increase in muscle weight stimulated by the weight training program. Weight gains of approximately one pound a week are about the best that most high school boys can anticipate with a well planned weight training and diet program.

Of critical importance in counseling young men regarding body building for sports and increasing muscle mass is to regularly monitor their weight gaining program to be sure that they are not increasing their level of body fat and to repeatedly counsel them about the dangers and ineffectiveness of drugs such as androgenic hormones, so-called steroids. In healthy young men these agents are ineffective in increasing muscle strength or muscle mass and can be associated with serious toxic side effects.

An important concern in dealing with young high school athletes who are interested in increasing their weight strength and endurance is to recognize whether or not the young athlete has arrived at a level of maturation at which his muscles can respond to increase work with increase in size and strength and a stage of maturity at which it is safe for him to subject his musculoskeletal system to the stresses of a regular weight training program. This is an important and commonly encountered concern for it is often the late maturing, tall, young man with immature, weak muscles and an immature skeletal system that is most anxious to develop more strength and endurance. This young man wants to get the basketball coach "off his back" who doesn't appreciate why this very tall boy can't hold his own against shorter and perhaps younger players who are more mature. Physicians are encouraged to inform coaches, parents and particularly young athletes of the normal maturation sequence experienced by young men as they acquire adult body size, weight, strength and endurance. Young men first grow in height. After experiencing their most rapid gains in height they will begin to increase significantly in weight through increases in muscle size. Then they will develop increases in strength and endurance. This normal sequence of growth events is regulated and controlled by the normal hormonal changes that occur during adolescence and is related directly to sexual maturation. Physicians monitor stages of adolescent development by grading stages of development of external genitalia and the development and distribution of body hair. Boys will not have a significant potential for developing increased muscle size and strength until approximately twelve to eighteen months after they have experienced their peak velocity in gains in height. At this stage testicular growth will have reached near adult size and a ready parameter of assessment is the distribution of genital hair which by this stage of maturation will have begun to appear on the inner aspects of the upper thigh. Prior to the appearance of genital hair on the inner aspects of the thigh young men should know that weight training, though it will yield modest increases in strength will not result in significant major gains in muscle mass and body weight.

The appropriate advice to the young man who is accepting the challenge of "making the team," but is a late maturer and is dissatisfied with his body size, muscle strength and endurance is to work on skills, participate in sports that are not dependent on strength and size. At the proper maturational stage he can become conscientious in pursuit of a well planned weight training and nutrition program. As young people make increasingly severe commitments to sport competition maturation assessment and counseling can be very important. Such counseling is an appropriate responsibility for team physician, trainer or coach at the high school level. Many tall, late maturing young men with real athletic potential have missed the opportunity of a rewarding sports experience by being pushed beyond his physical capabilities by parents and coaches whose performance expectations have been in relation to the boy's size without regard for his stage of maturity. The critical message here is not to involve these young men in regulated nutrition programs and weight training demands before their maturation status is such that they can be expected to experience reasonable benefits from the program.

In closing, a word about an area of nutrition advice the coach, trainer and health professional can profitably pass on to most athletes of most every age. This message may positively effect the nutritional well being and sports performance of many. It is most important for the high school athlete beginning to assume increasing responsibility for his or her own lifestyle and is the concern for not so much what these young people may be eating, but how and where they are experiencing their food intakes.

The nutrition interviews of the forty-eight varsity basketball players from the four Seattle high schools mentioned earlier provided some very disturbing information. More than a third of them stated that they never ate breakfast on school days and 17 of the forty-eight stated that they ate lunch irregularly. Candy ingestion one or more times a day was almost universal in this population. Twentytwo of the forty-eight, nearly half, stated that they had eaten their evening meal alone the night before the interview and frequently did so. It was of particular interest to find that although the schools involved included a very high income, suburban, all white school, a center city school in a low income area, with an all black team and two middle income neighborhood high schools, there was essentially no difference in the eating behavior of the members of the four different teams. If this is the way many of our young athletes are eating they can be helped with sound nutrition information from their coaches, trainers and the health professionals associated with their sports programs.

For the nearly ninety percent of Americans who can afford all the food they need, it is abundantly clear that the quality of their diet is directly proportional to the quality of the environment in which it is taken. For the family or the student athlete that can afford to feed themselves, the quality of their food intake is rarely a problem if they regularly eat in a nice place with some nice people. Meeting a girl friend, or boy friend, for lunch somewhere on the campus may do more to upgrade the quality of a student athlete's food intake than all the nutrition course work offered in the school. Eating alone and "on the run" is the surest way to eat poorly.

The critical nutrition message for the young athlete is to give nutrition and eating an appropriate priority in their lifestyle. Eat regularly with your family or good friends and take time to enjoy the experience of an adequate and healthy diet. The athlete's diet is both a major determinant of body composition and the source of energy to meet the demands of training and competition. How the athlete eats will make a difference in how he or she will perform on the field or court.

REFERENCES

1. Michener, J.A.: **Sports in America.** Random House, Inc., New York, 1976.

2. Bar-Or, O.,Climate and the Exercising Child, **Int. J. Sports Med.,** 1:53-65, 1980.

3. Shaffer, T.E., Smith, N.J. (ed.), **Sports Medicine for Children and Youth,** Ross Laboratories, Columbus, Ohio, 1979.

4. 10 STATE **Nutrition Survey,** Wash., D.C., Dept. W EW 1971.

5. Smith, N.J.: Food For Sport, Bull Publishing Co., Palo Alto, Calif., 1977.

6. Buskirk, E., Nutrition for the Athlete in Ryan, A.,Allman, F. (eds): Sports Medicine, Academic Press, New York, 1974.

7. Cook, J.D., Finch, C.A. and Smith, N.J., Evaluation of the Iron Status of a Population. **Blood** 48:449-456, 1976.

8. Finch, C.A., Miller, L.R.,Anamder, A.R., Persen, R., Seiler, K., and Mackler, B., Iron Deficiency in the Rat., **J. Clinic. Invest.,** 58:447-453, 1976.

9. Smith, N.J., Gaining and Losing Weight in Sports, **JAMA** 236:149-153, 1976.

Dietary Intake of the Older Athlete

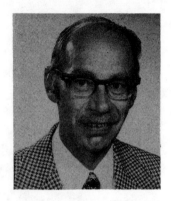

PETER D. WOOD, D.SC.

Adjunct Professor of Medicine, Stanford University School of Medicine. Deputy Director, Stanford Heart Disease Prevention Program. Author of many papers on cholesterol metabolism, heart disease prevention and exercise, and marathon runner. Member, American Institute of Nutrition and American Society for Clinical Nutrition.

For the purposes of this discussion the "older athlete" will be defined as a man or woman aged 40 or above who regularly engages in vigorous, aerobic sports. Before the "exercise explosion" of the past decade, such people were rare; but today some millions of individuals can probably be placed in this category in North America. However, the study of the nutritional requirements of the older athlete has accordingly been somewhat neglected until quite recently, and much remains to be learned. This contribution will first look briefly at the characteristics of a desirable diet for this group of very active people, and then consider the interaction of vigorous activity, dietary intake and health in older men and women.

OPTIMAL NUTRITION FOR THE OLDER ATHLETE

This subject can be considered from two points of view: the long-term nutritonal requirements for general good health and prevention (or at least postponement) of the major chronic diseases such as heart disease, stroke and cancer; and also the optimal composition of the diet for short-term, effective athletic performance. The desirable long-term diet for optimal health in the older athlete is very little, if at all, different from the desirable diet for the younger athlete, or indeed for the population in general.

Opinions on the nature of this widely-applicable desirable diet range over a spectrum, with some extreme recommendations; but the consensus of informed scientific opinion is probably best crystallized in the recommendations of the Senate Select Committee on Nutrition and Human Needs in their Dietary Goals for the United States[1]. In brief, this diet is composed of 30 percent of total calories as fat, 10-15% as protein and 55-60% as carbohydrate. The fat should contain no more than 10% of total calories as saturated fat, and 10% as polyunsaturated fat (e.g. vegetable oil). Cholesterol intake in the diet should be restricted to less than 300 mg per day. Sugar (sucrose) should be less than 10% of total calories, and salt intake should be below 5 grams per day. Dietary fiber should be increased. This widely applicable prescription is not extreme, is consistent with a generally palatable and acceptable diet and almost certainly will improve the national health with respect to several chronic diseases, notably heart disease. Since older athletes, such as runners, are not entirely immune to atherosclerosis and its unfortunate consequences[2,3], these dietary goals are clearly desirable for this group as much as for any other.

The major characteristic of the diet of the older athlete is its high calorie content. As we shall discuss later, very active people eat more than sedentary people. For instance, a very active older woman tennis player may require almost twice the caloric intake of a very sedentary woman[4]. This feature of the older athlete's diet relates to the question of whether very active people—young or old need increased amounts of specific nutrients, such as protein, vitamins and minerals. The short answer is that such individuals do require modestly increased intakes of such nutrients, and that they automatically get them by virtue of their increased intake of food in general. There is also a widespread belief that athletes, perhaps older athletes in particular, will benefit from greatly increased amounts of specific nutrients, for instance total protein, vitamin C, vitamin E and lecithin, to mention a few popular favorites. In a recent survey of 253 male runners aged 50-64, reporting an average of 30 miles of running per week (members of the Fifty-Plus Runners Association), 60-70% reported taking

TABLE 1. Reported Use of Vitamins, Minerals and Other Supplements Among Male Runners Aged 50-64.

Supplement	Percentage Reporting Use		
	Age 50-54 (n=133)	Age 55-59 (n=81)	Age 60-64 (n=39)
Vitamin A	5	10	10
Vitamin B	18	22	26
Vitamin C	43	43	41
Vitamin D	2	5	5
Vitamin E	23	29	31
Multiple vitamins	37	37	46
Any vitamin supplement	59	61	69
Zinc	7	9	13
Calcium	4	6	3
Dolomite	3	7	8
Magnesium	2	4	0
Potassium	2	2	3
Selenium	2	1	0
Lecithin	7	9	13
Brewer's yeast	6	2	5
Bee pollen	4	9	8
Garlic	2	5	0
Wheat germ	2	1	3
Kelp	1	1	3

supplemental vitamins, and a sizeable proportion reported taking a variety of mineral and other supplements (Table 1). The scientific literature, however, provides very little basis for a requirement for relatively large supplements of these dietary components; and there are virtually no well-designed studies indicating that any long-term nutritional supplement significantly improves athletic performance at any age in normal individuals. It should be noted that few well-designed studies have been performed in this difficult area, and so the possibility exists that certain supplements may prove to be beneficial in the future. There is some evidence that individuals consuming larger amounts of dietary carotene are less likely to develop certain cancers than those consuming smaller amounts[5]. The relationship of intake of certain vitamins and minerals, and their plasma concentrations, to risk of developing cancer is a very active research area at this time.

In summary, there is little evidence to suggest that the long-term diet of the older athlete should be very different from that of the normal, but sedentary, individual, except that the caloric content must reflect the increased energy expenditure of the athlete. However, the diet of the older athlete (and of the American population in general) would be improved by a move towards the prudent dietary goals set by a number of expert groups, for instance those of the Senate Select Committee.

Dietary intake in the short-term, in relation to athletic performance, does ideally differ in some respects for the older athlete compared to the sedentary individual. Again, the major principles are not different as between younger and older athletes.

The amount and type of food consumed shortly before an athletic event should be determined on the basis of comfort and experience. For events involving running, most older athletes prefer to have eaten lightly or not at all within the previous 4-6 hours. Lighter, liquid foods are often prefered to heavier, solid foods. The pre-event consumption of large amounts of "quick energy" foods, such as glucose, has not proved to be beneficial in the endurance sports, although glucose may be beneficial to performance in the later stages of endurance events such as marathon running and long-distance cycling.

A vital short-term dietary component for all athletes is water. The importance of performing in an adequately hydrated state is extreme, especially in the longer events, and especially when climatic conditions are hot and/or humid. Water is the one item "taken by mouth" that can become in short supply during an athletic event lasting some hours. It must be replaced, at least partially during the event. If this is not done, the risk of serious dehydration with resulting discomfort, rise in body core temperature, confusion, collapse and sometimes death is always present. Heat damage due to dehydration is one of the most serious hazards for athletes of all ages. This is well illustrated by the annual scene at the end of the Boston Marathon race, where several hundred apparently exhausted and dehydrated runners are routinely rehydrated by administration of intravenous fluids, after which they rapidly recover and go their way. Both individual athletes and competition climatic conditions vary in subtle and little understood ways with respect to risk of serious dehydration. The solution is adequate hydration before, during and after any event with a sustained high energy output, especially those lasting for more than 30 minutes. Older and younger athletes should accustom themselves to drinking more water than their thirst dictates, and adjusting their water intake during the event to match the climatic conditions. Athletic drinks with high glucose contents (approximately 5%) are undesirable, since stomach emptying time tends to be increased, making the water content relatively less available. There is some discussion about the value of lower concentrations of glucose, and of added minerals such as sodium and potassium. Such low-glucose drinks with added minerals do no harm and may be beneficial in endurance events; but water remains the one vital component that must be replaced.

The use of salt tablets on hot days has mercifully decreased and should be abandoned entirely in normal North American conditions. In the long-term, the average diet provides more than enough sodium for older athletes—and often too much; in the short-term, the dehydrated athlete needs water, not salt.

The practice of "carbohydrate loading" is popular with endurance athletes of all ages. This pre-event technique involves an exhausting bout of exercise to considerably deplete muscle glycogen, followed by some days on a high-protein, low-carbohydrate diet to continue the depletion, with a final few days on a high carbohydrate diet to produce a "super-high" muscle glycogen content just prior to the big event. The high-protein, low-carbohydrate phase is often unpleasant for the athlete, and may be hazardous in extreme circumstances: it is often eliminated by athletes who go straight to the high carbohydrate phase. There is no question that this loading process tends to increase muscle glycogen concentration. Many athletes, including older athletes, report apparently beneficial effects on performance, and there is some scientific evidence to support this. However, it should be borne in mind that adequate muscle glycogen content is only one of a series of requirements for good endurance performance. If glycogen content is the weakest link in the chain, then carbohydrate loading may produce significant improvement. However, if deficiencies in the cardiovascular system, or in mechanical efficiency are the weakest links, then loading may produce disappointing results. Trial-and-error appears to be the only way to judge the value of this procedure in an individual case.

A final short-term dietary component that has gained some popularity is alcohol, especially beer. Although there is some evidence that long-term moderate alcohol intake is associated with reduced risk of coronary heart disease[6], there is no evidence that beer consumption during endurance events such as the marathon has any advantages over the consumption of similar volumes of pure water; and for many athletes the carbonation of beer is a source of gastric discomfort during exercise.

THE INTERACTION OF VIGOROUS ACTIVITY, DIET AND HEALTH IN OLDER ATHELTES

The process of growing older in America is usually accompanied by a series of changes related to dietary intake and exercise level, all of which are associated with deterioration of either health, performance or appearance. The way in which the older athlete copes with this statistically normal evolution beyond age 40 will be considered under several headings.

Decreased Aerobic Capacity

Cross-sectional population surveys indicate a decreasing fitness level, measured in terms of maximal oxygen uptake, with advancing age in the United States. However, individuals who remain aerobically active into middle and older age are able to slow down this process considerably, and those who continue to compete at a high level show a much slower decline[7]. Many studies have shown substantial cross-sectional differences in aerobic capacity of older exercisers of both sexes compared with sedentary controls[4,8]. Training studies (e.g.,[9]) have shown that a progressive exercise conditioning program in older sedentary individuals predictably improves aerobic capacity to a gratifying extent. It is therefore up to the individual to a considerable degree whether he or she becomes progressively less fit, or maintains fitness into older age.

Increased Body Fat, Decreased Lean Body Mass

The typical American gains body weight as fat steadily from age 20 to age 50, by which time some 30 pounds of extra fat has been accumulated. Muscle or lean body mass is typically lost from middle age onwards. Numerous studies have shown that very active older individuals of either sex are relatively lean compared to their sedentary peers[4,8]. Furthermore, training programs among older, sedentary individuals invariably lead to loss of body fat if they are reasonably vigorous and maintained for at least several months[10]. As shown in Table 2, some 85% of male runners aged 50-64 report weight loss since starting a running program. As with aerobic

SPECIAL PROBLEMS

TABLE 2. Reported Body Weight Change Since Starting to Run in Male Runners Aged 50-64.

Age (No of men)	Per Cent Reporting:		
	Weight Loss	**No Change**	**Weight Gain**
50-54 (133)	86	13	0
55-59 (81)	84	12	4
60-64 (39)	84	16	0

TABLE 3. Total Recorded Caloric Intake and Experience of Coronary Heart Disease (CHD) in Men in Four Prospective Studies.

Study (Reference)	Mean Daily Caloric Intake	
	No CHD	**Myocardial Infarction or CHD Death**
United Kingdom bank employees and busmen (16)	2869	2656**
Framingham (17)	2622	2369*
Puerto Rico (17)	2395	2223*
Honolulu (17)	2319	2149**

*$p < 0.05$; **$p < 0.01$

capacity, the inexorable decline in muscle mass with age in the sedentary individual can be slowed by continued regular physical activity[11]. It is thus true that body composition, and hence appearance, is under the older individual's personal control to a considerable degree. Many older joggers have discoverd the truth—often disputed in earlier times—that increased physical activity really does help to control body weight.

Decreased Caloric Intake

It has been regarded as paradoxical by some that the increased fatness typically occurring with aging in America is accompanied by decreased total daily caloric intake[12]. In fact, many studies indicate that more obese people tend to eat less, rather than more, than thinner people[13]. The caloric cost of increased physical activity is, of course, the key to understanding these superficially paradoxical findings. Cross-sectional surveys of dedicated older runners[14] and older tennis players[4] of both sexes, and of suitable sedentary control groups, have indicated daily caloric intakes 40-80% greater on a weight-adjusted basis for the active people. A Stanford study of 14 initially sedentary men aged 36-54 who completed a 2-year running program (average 12 miles run per week) indicated an increased recorded calorie intake of about 260 calories per day whilst running[15]. On the usual basis of a caloric cost of 100 calories per mile run, the mean daily increase should have been about 170 calories for this group, so that the true caloric cost of running exceeds 100 calories per mile, or other unrecorded energy-consuming activities were performed by the participants, or both.

The conclusion from such studies is that here again the very active older person resembles more the younger person, and the usual age-related decline in calorie consumption is abolished or slowed. There are several noteworthy consequences of this for the older athlete. First, the older athlete can maintain the previously-noted desirable body composition while enjoying a high caloric intake. He or she is usually freed from the preoccupation with calorie counting that afflicts the average older person. Second, since a higher total food intake is usually accompanied by increased vitamin and mineral intake, the chances of deficiency of these micronutrients in older people who exercise are reduced. Lastly, there is an interesting association between higher daily caloric intakes and reduced future risk of heart attack in men, as shown in at least four prospective population studies (Table 3). It may be speculated that the higher caloric intakes reflect higher mean levels of physical activity in the "protected" groups.

Changed Plasma Lipoprotein Pattern

The extensive population surveys of the Lipid Research Clinics[18] have indicated age-related changes in plasma lipoprotein patterns that have been associated with increased risk of coronary heart disease. In men, plasma triglycerides and very-low-density lipoprotein (VLDL) cholesterol concentrations increase with age, the atherogenic low-density lipoprotein (LDL) cholesterol level also increases, and the level of the possibly anti-atherogenic high-density lipoprotein (HDL) cholesterol remains relatively constant with age. Changes in women with age are similar, except that HDL-cholesterol concentration tends to rise. A number of studies have shown that the older aerobic athlete maintains a relatively desirable lipoprotein pattern, with respect to risk of heart disease, in spite of his or her age. The older male athlete typically has a pattern (low VLDL- and LDL-cholesterol, high HDL-cholesterol) that is characteristic of young women. The Stanford training study in 14 initially sedentary men[15] showed an improvement after two years of running an average of 12 miles per week in the important heart disease risk indicator, total cholesterol concentration ÷ HDL-cholesterol (ratio of 4.46 at baseline significantly reduced to 3.86 after two years).

Increased Risk of Coronary Heart Disease

Risk of developing coronary heart disease increases with age in the United States. Aging itself is generally considered to have a strong, independent and unavoidable influence on risk. But many of the remaining "risk factors" are favorably influenced by the vigorous lifestyle of the older athlete:

■ Improved plasma lipoprotein pattern.

■ Maintenance of desirable body weight.

■ Aeorbic fitness maintained at high level.

■ Relatively high caloric intake.

■ Absence or low level of cigarette smoking.

The presence of elevated blood pressure constitutes a further powerful risk factor. Resting blood pressure may be somewhat lowered in older athletes by virtue of their leanness; and blood pressure under conditions of exercise stress is clearly reduced by exercise training.

It may be concluded that the dietary and exercise habits of the older athlete favor a considerably reduced risk of coronary heart disease. But it should also be noted that an improvement in the qualitative nature of the diet selected by the older athlete, as discussed earlier, will further improve his already reduced risk of coronary disease via the effect upon plasma lipids and blood pressure.

Other Problems of Aging

Two other diet-related conditions frequently encountered in older people appear to be favorably influenced by the dietary and exercise habits of the older athlete.

The inexorable loss of bone mineral, notably calcium, with aging, especially in postmenopausal women, can lead to pronounced osteoporsis and bone fractures. The older athlete is favored from two viewpoints: regular exercise appears to retard mineral loss from bones; and the increased caloric intake of the older exerciser is likely to be accompanied by an increased calcium intake.

Constipation is another concomitant of older age of many Americans. Apparently this annoying condition is relatively rare among older athletes, as judged from a recent survey of the Fifty-Plus Runners Association. This may be a result of the mechanical action of the athletic performance itself; but in addition the higher daily food intake, with an increased fiber content, may contribute.

In summary, the increased energy output and the concomitant increased energy intake of the older athlete appear to provide several substantial health advantages. Two major dietary recommendations are made to further improve the already favorable health outlook of the older athlete:

- Short-term: maintain adequate hydration.

- Long-term: move toward a more prudent diet.

ACKNOWLEDGEMENTS

The author appreciates the cooperation of members of the Fifty-Plus Runners Association. This work was supported in part by NIH grant No. HL 24462.

REFERENCES

1. Dietary Goals for the United States. **Report of the Select Committee on Nutrition and Human Needs, U.S. Senate.** Second edition, December 1977

2. Thompson, P.D., M.P. Stern, P. Williams, K. Duncan, W.L. Haskell, and P.D. Wood. Death during jogging or running: A study of 18 cases. **JAMA** 242:1265-1267, 1979.

3. Thompson, P.D., E.J. Funk, R.A. Carleton, and W.Q. Sturner. Incidence of death during jogging in Rhode Island from 1975 through 1980. **JAMA** 247:2535-2538, 1982.

4. Vodak, P.A., P.D. Wood, W.L. Haskell, and P.T. Williams. HDL-cholesterol and other plasma lipid and lipoprotein concentrations in middle-aged male and female tennis players. **Metabolism** 29:745-752, 1980.

5. Peto, R., R. Doll, J.D. Buckley, and M.B. Sporn. Can dietary beta-carotene materially reduce human cancer rates? **Nature** 290:201-208, 1981.

6. Castelli, W.P., J.T. Doyle, T. Gordon, et al. Alcohol and blood lipids: the Cooperative Lipoprotein Phenotyping Study. **Lancet** 2:153-155, 1977.

7. Pollock, M.L., C. Foster, J. Rod, J. Hare, and D.H. Schmidt. Ten year follow-up on the aerobic capacity of champion master's track athletes. **Med. Sci. Sports Exercise** 14:105, 1982. (Abstract)

8. Wood, P.D. and W.L. Haskell. The effect of exercise on plasma high density lipoproteins. **Lipids** 14:417-427, 1979.

9. Wood, P.D., W.L. Haskell, S.N. Blair, et al. Increased exercise level and plasma lipoprotein concentrations. A one-year, randomized, controlled study in sedentary, middle-aged men. **Metabolism** 1982 (in press).

10. Williams, P.T., P.D. Wood, W.L. Haskell, and K. Vranizan. The effects of running mileage and duration on plasma lipoprotein levels. **JAMA** 247:2674-2679, 1982.

11. Lewis, S., W.L. Haskell, H. Klein, J. Halpern, and P.D. Wood. Prediction of body composition in habitually active middle-aged men. **J. Appl. Physiol.** 39:221-225, 1975.

12. Friend, B., L. Page, and R. Marston. Food consumption patterns in the United States: 1909-13 to 1976. **In: Nutrition, Lipids and Coronary Heart Disease,** R.I. Levy, B.M. Rifkind, B.H. Dennis, and N.D. Ernst (Eds.) New York: Raven, 1979, pp. 489-522.

13. Keen H., B.H. Thomas, R.J. Jarrett, et al. Nutrient intake, adiposity, and diabetes. **Brit. Med. J.** 2:1307-1314, 1977.

14. Blair, N.S., N.M. Ellsworth, W.L. Haskell, M.P. Stern, J.W. Farquihar, and P.D. Wood. Comparison of nutrient intake in middle-aged men and women runners and controls. **Med. Sci. Sports Exercise** 13:310-315, 1981.

15. Wood, P.D., W.L. Haskell, R.B. Terry, P.H. Ho, and S.N. Blair. Effects of a two-year running program on plasma lipoproteins, body fat and dietary intake in initially sedentary men. **Med. Sci. Sports Exercise** 14:104, 1982. (Abstract)

16. Morris, J.N., J.W. Marr, and D.G. Clayton. Diet and heart: a postscript. **Brit. Med. J.** 2:1307-1314, 1977.

17. Gordon, T., A. Kagan, M. Garcia-Palmieri, et al. Diet and its relation to coronary heart disease in three populations. **Circulation** 63:500-515, 1981.

18. Heiss, G., I. Tamir, C.E. Davis, et al. Lipoprotein-cholesterol distributions in selected North American populations: The Lipid Research Clinics Program Prevalence Study. **Circulation** 61:302-315, 1980.

Summary

Controversies developed during the discussion of Dr. Pate's presentation on sports anemia, principally centered around the three probable reasons he gave for low iron storage and risk of anemia: inadequate dietary iron, low absorption of iron from the digestive tract, and high rates of iron loss. It is clear from the Hanes Study and the Nationwide Food Consumption Survey II that dietary intake of iron for adults is frequently inadequate when compared to the iron RDA. This is particularly true for women between the ages of 12 and 50, whose intakes average only 58-64% of their RDA's for iron. These figures are consistent with data showing an average of 6 mg iron per 1000 kcals of food consumed, given that the U.S. averages for caloric intake are estimated at 2400 kcals and 1600 kcals for women. Theoretically, athletes may be at unusually high risk for anemia, in part due to the fad diets used by many athletes, which increase the risk of inadequate dietary iron.

The recent work of Cook (**J. Cereal Food World 26:667, 1981**) is one of a series of studies which indicate that even though the dietary iron may be in the food, it may not be adequately absorbed. This may be due in part to phytates and fiber, but the effect is quite dramatic even with the usual cup of tea or coffee. On the other hand, it appears that ascorbic acid taken with the meal may help increase the iron absorption of non-heme food iron. The early work of Yoshimura (**Nutr. Rev. 28:251, 1970**) and Williamson (**Physician and Sports Medicine 9:73, 1981**) imply that athletes may be subjected to extraordinarily high rates of iron loss, due to increased destruction of erythrocytes during strenuous muscular exercise. All of these factors may contribute to reduced iron levels in athletes during prolonged seasons of training and competition.

There was a debate of what constitutes a correct measure of adequate iron. There was a general consensus that hemoglobin levels in the studies conducted on athletes do not indicate that athletes in general are more anemic than non-exercising individuals; measures of just hemoglobin may not be the answer. Serum ferritin levels and iron stores should be measured over long periods of time to determine the drain of iron from the body. The simple total iron binding capacity is not always a true indicator of the bone marrow iron storage.

As summarized by Jack Henenauer, U.C.S.D., reporting on some of his own work, when women with normal hemoglobin levels were subjected to a mild exercise program, "you generally do not see much movement in hematological status. However, significant improvement in their overall aerobic performance was also not exhibited." Studies of intense activity, on the other hand, tend to show different results, and prolonged intense activity may be where the real cause of sports anemia lies. As observed by Runyan and Puhl, there is a decline in hemoglobin values after a few weeks of mild exercise when people with normal hemoglobin values are subjected to an exercise program. This is probably not just a hemodilution factor but, in fact, a new synthesis of red blood cells with a smaller than normal amount of hemoglobin. This, in fact, implies iron redistribution. This effect is usually seen over a period of a few weeks after the exercise program has begun.

It may be that this type of iron anemia is best assessed **not** by reference to a population standard of hemoglobin value, but rather, through measurements in conjunction with intakes of increased amounts of iron. Where there is an increase in the heme level, the person should be considered anemic—no change in heme status would indicate he is at capacity.

Finally, as reported by Ohira and Edgerton (**Handbook of Nutritional Requirements in a Functional Context,** Vol. II, Edited by M. Rechcigl, CRC Press, Boca Raton, FL, 1981), although hemoglobin levels do not always rise when iron supplements are given, it has been demonstrated that iron supplementation induces significant bradycardia and increased physical work performance in iron deficient, anemic and also normal individuals. Heart rate at submaximal workload decrease, and VO_2 max increased, in iron supplementally trained females versus non-supplementally trained females. Ericcson (**Acta. Med. Scand. 188:361, 1970**) also found that healthy elderly subjects showed increased physical work capacity on iron supplementation, even though hemoglobin status was unchanged. The fact that hemoglobin status did not change in these studies suggests some improvement of tissue iron metabolism due to iron intake. The mechanism of such supplemental iron on physiological function is unclear.

The presentation by Dr. Leon provided a comprehensive review of the conditions and nature of diabetes. He also discussed in considerable detail diabetic management and, particularly, the role of exercise as a contributory factor in the management of this condition. The subject of abnormal platelet adhesiveness was discussed in relation to the diabetic. While it is agreed that diabetics do have abnormal platelet adhesiveness, there is no evidence presently that exercise will actually reverse this condition.

Platelet adhesiveness is often caused by hyperinsulin anemia, which can, in fact, contribute to an abnormal effect. In this case, simple reduction of insulin would be the appropriate remedy. Theoretically, however, the dilution factor caused by exercise, with resultant increased plasma volume, should help reduce blood viscosity. This, as a secondary mechanism, would reduce the perceived platelet adhesiveness.

Various questions arose concerning how the diabetic knows when his glucose levels are at a safe level before a particular exercise event. It soon became apparent that this varies from individual to individual, as well as with the degree of exertion. Studies of individuals who have glucose levels between 200 mg/deciliter and 300 mg/deciliter have not been documented, primarily because such levels would not be received as safe for humans in a clinical study. In a specific case of a diabetic class marathon runner, the individual's own rule of thumb was to be spilling +3 in his urine before the start of an event of this intensity. This was apparently adequate assurance for him that his blood levels were high enough; but this was for an elite runner, and should not be used as a rule of thumb for every individual.

It is most important, when an individual first initiates intense physical exercise, that he work closely with a physician and trainer to develop a planned, rational program, one step at a time. The most important objective is to prevent ketosis. It was also pointed out that the use of home glucose monitoring instruments is becoming more and more commonplace, due to their simplicity and convenience. Such instruments definitely can help the diabetic athlete assess his or her sugar levels, and quantitatively estimate safe ranges for intensive exercise. In general, these instruments are more accurate than urine analysis. Generally speaking, a sugar level of between 100-120 mg per deciliter is a good level at which to start exercise but, once again, intensity and duration of the exercise need to be worked out by the individual and his physician.

It must also be reemphasized that fluids are just as important for the diabetic as they are for the "normal" athlete, and need to be replaced. The general recommendation that body fluids be replenished during an endurance event with a solution of 2.5% glucose or less is equally appropriate for the diabetic athlete.

It was also suggested that, where practical, diabetics should consider a carbohydrate snack at intervals during long-term exercise. Whether or not fructose is better than glucose in such snacks and drinks was a subject of much discussion. The American Dietetic Association has chosen not to make any recommendations regarding which monosaccharide is better, simply because evidence is lacking. Theoretically, fructose could be the better of the two, but all participants felt that research evidence is still needed.

Finally, to prepare for aerobic events of long duration, carbohydrate loading at calorie levels of 60 percent or more of carbohydrates, particularly in the form of starch, would certainly serve the needs of the diabetic, and play a dual role: The use of complex carbohydrates allows a gradual perfusion of glucose into the blood, while maintaining the muscle glycogen stores.

Dr. Smith provided a comprehensive summary of the nutritional problems faced by the young athlete preparing for competition. The major nutritional concern of any young child is to compensate for increased caloric expenditure with an adequate supply of nutritionally sound food. The major issue that developed in the discussion of this presentation applies to all young children and young adults; that is, how to provide the growing body with a sound nutritional format. As pointed out in the Hanes and Ten State Studies, besides energy, children 3-8 years of age are having some difficulty meeting the USRDA requirements for iron, calcium, magnesium, and many of the B vitamins. It was mentioned that young males from a poverty setting may be having a greater problem in meeting their needs than females from similar areas.

Just as important, however, is the need to educate the young and instill good eating habits in them at an early age. The concepts of controlling weight, lowering sodium and sugar intake, increasing fiber consumption, and altering dietary intake of fats to levels of approximately 30% of total calories are good health goals for all young people, whether athletes or not.

Dr. Wood's presentation elucidated the fact that sensible nutrition, whether for the young, mature, or older athlete, is the best recommendation any nutritionist can provide. Guidelines recommended by the Senate Select Committee on Nutrition and Human Needs and supported by other respected groups would include 10-15% of total calories from protein, 55-60% from carbohydrates and less than 30% from fat. The most recent available dietary intake data show that the typical diet pattern of most Americans is quite different from these recommendations. The Nationwide Food Consumption Survey of 1977-1978 shows that individuals 23 to 50 years of age had a caloric distribution of approximately 17% from protein, 43% from fat, and 40% from carbohydrate. Furthermore, certain groups did not appear to obtain the USRDA of vitamin B_6, calcium, iron, and magnesium. Dr. Wood's research found that men runners' dietary intake consisted of 14% protein, 40% carbohydrate, 41% fat and 5% alcohol, which is not much different than the intake of the average American adult.

With regard to lean muscle mass, it is Dr. Wood's conclusion that there is no physiologic reason for a decrease in muscle mass with age, unless the older person exercises less.

A question still remaining to be answered, however, is whether there is an increased nutrient need for the older athlete, especially given that metabolic activity and absorptive capacity may decrease.

Concluding Comments

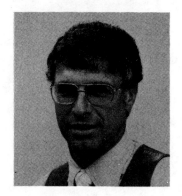

PAUL SALTMAN, PH.D.

Professor of Biology, University of California, San Diego.
Author of "America and the Future of Man" for the National Endowment for the Humanities, and consultant to the National Science Foundation and the Academy of Sciences. Recipient of Research Career Development Award from National Institutes of Health. Numerous publications and research projects in the field of iron biochemistry.

One of the most important topics related to nutritional determinants in athletic performance has not been discussed at this Conference. In some ways it is the heart of the matter. In other ways it is irrational and ephemeral. That topic is the metaphysics of food and diet and how what we eat profoundly affects our athletic performance.

This symposium has focused our attention on the science of nutrition. Rigorous and reproducible experiments have laid the foundation for the formulation of complete, semi-synthetic Total Parenteral Nutrition. No one admonishes the patient with an indwelling catheter dripping a life-giving emulsion into his blood or stomach "to choose wisely from the four basic food groups". Clearly we know the human body's requirements for water, calories, carbohydrate, essential amino acids, vitamins, minerals, and trace elements.

But, nutrition for all of us is more than a bag of nutrients. Nutrition transcends the complex biochemical and physiological metabolic panorama of our bodies' structure and function. Nutrition is food. Nutrition is what we eat, how much we eat, when and with whom we eat, and what beliefs we share regarding the food we eat. There is an essential metascience of nutrition which is inextricably entwined with the science of nutrition.

Nowhere is this relationship more clearly observed than at the "training table" of a powerful football team, in the sweating and starving off of precious pounds by a jockey or wrestler trying to "make" weight, the carbohydrate-loading of a marathon runner, or the swilling of jars and bottles of pills, potions and concoctions of bee pollen, wheat germ oil, and honey . . . or for that matter, whatever the current fad or rage of a particular sport might be . . . by an athlete trying in every way to achieve a "personal best".

Our interest is not primarily concerned with the world champion. We must direct our attention to each and every man and woman, boy and girl, who is an active participant in sport. The champion epitomizes the ultimate in sport, the culmination and integration of genes and environment, endowed gifts and acquired skills, and . . . above all . . . a will to win. That champion must call upon every possible nutritional advantage to operate his or her body at ultimate performance. No less important from the standpoint of health and performance are the nutritional needs of the recreational or competitive athlete. The situation is analagous to the maintenance and tuning of automobiles. There is a difference between the needs of a race car and those of a street vehicle. But, the similarities for fuel, lubrication, spark plugs, tires, etc., are more impressive, than are the differences.

There is so much nonsense in the popular literature about what foods provide the best source of energy for sport. Drs. Butterfield and Costill clarified this issue. There are both short- and long-term issues. The short-term effects of immediate dietary consumption before athletic activity include stomach emptying time, digestibility, and utilizability. The notion that different foods or nutrients provide "different" calories is both mythic and false. The long-term effects of being assured optimal amounts of stored carbohydrate as glycogen in the muscle is of fundamental importance. To maintain optimal oxidative metabolism, carbohydrate must provide the primary molecules for the Krebs cycle. Fats, as fatty acids, are not gluconeogenic. Proteins, as amino acids, can provide glycolytic intermediates, but at a greater metabolic cost. Thus, the practice of glycogen loading muscle cells by a properly planned regimen of exercise and high starch/sugar diet can provide an "edge" for the trained endurance athlete.

Salt and water balance are frequently ignored or poorly understood by athletes and coaches. There are two aspects to this problem. The first is the loss of fluids during strenuous activity via perspiration and respiration. Replacement of these fluids is essential both during and after exercise. Magic elixars with power-punch names are little more effective than water, juice, milk or other less exotic liquids. The second is the deliberate loss of water via lowered intake, increased salivary and urine flow, and sweating encountered while trying to "make" weight. These practices involve upsetting both fluid, electrolyte and nutritional intake. Serious long-term consequences are attendant to these practices, particularly in high school athletes during their growing years.

I am reminded of many shibboleths regarding drinking water during basketball games, or the evils of milk consumed before events leading to muscle cramping that have now, fortunately, been dispelled. I remember one high school coach who warned us of the evils of lactic acid causing muscle cramps if we drank milk. He never knew the difference between lactose and lactic acid, much less the metabolic relation between them.

Too many claims have been made for the wonders of mega-vitamin and mega-mineral supplements for athletes. Too few if any reasonable double-blind studies have been made using trained athletes to test their effectiveness. Many years ago at the University of Southern California I carried out experiments with their great track team which indicated that placebos were as effective as supplements in fully trained athletes. When the trackmen were "forced" by experiment to run without the "Super

Power Pill", their performance was impaired. There is a delicate and potent balance of mind and muscle.

However, the use of rational supplements, i.e., one or two RDA's of known required vitamins and minerals might well be encouraged. It is increasingly difficult in our complex, varied, and processed food chain, not to mention the bizarre fashion in which we function as family units in the preparation and consumption of meals, to be assured of adequate nourishment. Strenuous exercise can alter the rate of loss of some trace elements, particularly zinc and copper. No one has accurately measured metabolic losses of vitamins under severe muscular activity. It is an experiment whose time has come.

Body weight and composition are important parameters of health and performance. Too often there is confusion regarding total body mass and relative body composition. Increasingly we take notice of the percent of fat, the volume of fluid and muscle mass. Our intent is to "shape" optimal bodies for particular events. We train and feed with malice and forethought. It is no wonder that coaches, physicians and physiologists are striving to find the optimal training and feeding programs.

There was a time when sport was for boys and men. We've come a long way, baby! Not only are girls and women, but also young and old, normal and handicapped, and healthy and diseased, encouraged to participate actively and strenuously in sport. There are attendant nutritional problems. Young children are frequently carried mentally and physically far beyond their reasonable capacity. Too much stress on winning, too little encouragement for the growth and development of healthy minds and bodies. Dr. Smith revealed what most of us knew but did not want to believe. Among high school athletes from rich and poor families, little or no attention is paid to nutritional needs. Life-styles of "three squares a day" of the "basic four" are replaced by on-the-run potatoe chips, donuts, and soft drinks offering calories and water galore, but little else. Coaches and physicians working with the young athletes and their parents must take an active role in eating practices.

Thanks to modern medicine and enlightened nutritional practices, it is now possible to permit a diabetic to participate fully in competitive sport. So, too, have various handicapped individuals been encouraged to flex their minds and muscles in sport. Extra care and caution must be taken to ensure that these efforts are within reasonable physical bounds and that attention is given to specific nutritional needs.

The "baby boom" is over. Gray and graying panthers are running, jumping, swimming, skiing, hitting various sized balls with various shaped rackets. It is wondrous to contemplate. There is an increasing awareness the relationship among the factors of age, nutrition, and exercise as determinants of health and constructive longevity. As the body ages, particular attention must be paid to those systems, such as circulation, skeletal and excretory, where diet plays a profound role. No magic diet, be it from Beverly Hills or Scarsdale, or carrying the name of Pritikin or Atkins, is nearly as effective as a rational, calorically balanced, nutritionally complete diet developed to an individual's taste and metabolic needs.

Each of us cherishes unique and particular notions of what tastes good, makes us feel good, and is good for us. Those notions are a far cry from the contents of the bag containing Total Parenteral Nutrition. Our challenge is to pursue relentlessly a better understanding of the scientific basis of nutrition and at the same time to exhalt in the joys and pleasures of manifesting our athletic prowess. We must optimize our physical and metaphysical human potential with its energy and nutrients derived from the diverse and delicious cuisine spread upon the dining tables of our lives.